Beat Hammer

Orbital Fractures

Herrn Dr. Weitisch
freundschaftlich
zugeeignet.

Aarau 30.8.95

B. Hammer

Beat Hammer

Orbital Fractures
Diagnosis
Operative Treatment
Secondary Corrections

Foreword by Paul Tessier, Paris

Hogrefe & Huber Publishers
Seattle · Toronto · Bern · Göttingen

Library of Congress Cataloging-in-Publication Data

Hammer, Beat
Orbital Fractures – Diagnosis, Operative Treatment, Secondary Corrections

available via the Library of Congress Marc Database under the

LC Catalog Card Number 94-073194

Canadian Cataloguing in Publication Data

Hammer, Beat, 1951–
  Orbital fractures : diagnosis, operative treatment, secondary corrections

Includes bibliographical references and index.
ISBN 0-88937-139-3

1. Eye-sockets – Fractures. 2. Eye-sockets – Surgery. I. Title.

RD527.E94E35   1995   617.7'8059   C94-932837-5

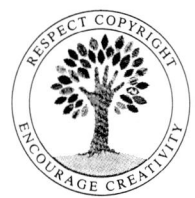

ISBN 0-88937-139-3
Hogrefe & Huber Publishers, Seattle • Toronto • Bern • Göttingen
ISBN 3-8017-0785-2
Hogrefe & Huber Publishers, Göttingen • Bern • Seattle • Toronto

© 1995 by Hogrefe & Huber Publishers
USA: P.O. Box 2487, Kirkland, WA 98083-2487,
                 Phone (206) 820-1500, Fax (206) 823-8324
CANADA: 12 Bruce Park Avenue, Toronto, Ontario M4P 2S3
                 Phone (416) 482-6339
SWITZERLAND: Länggass-Strasse 76, CH-3000 Bern 9
                 Phone (031) 300-4500, Fax (031) 300-4590
GERMANY: Rohnsweg 25, D-37085 Göttingen
                 Phone (0551) 496090, Fax (0551) 4960988

No part of this book may be reproduced, stored in a retrieval system, or transmitted, in any form or by any means, electronic, mechanical, photocopying, microfilming, recording or otherwise, without the written permission from the publisher.

Typeset by Joseph A. Smith, SATZSPIEGEL, Göttingen
Printed and bound in Germany

Foreword

The eyes and the surrounding areas are perhaps the most fascinating feature of the human face. But whether blue, brown, or green, our eyes are poorly protected cerebral sensors. And people may be able to live without smell, without hearing, and without taste, but they cannot survive alone without vision in what is essentially a hostile environment.

Noses can be distorted, jaws displaced, and foreheads plagiocephalic, without necessarily detracting from the beauty of the whole. But however beautiful its form, the true charm of a human face lies in two components: the gaze and glance of the eyes, and a smile spreading from the lips to the eyelids. Furthermore, eyes come in pairs, and so the loss of vision in one eye is often less cruel than the permanent torture of double vision which often results in amblyopia.

The orbital region and the ocular adnexae exist only to protect the eye and visual function. Surgical corrections or reconstructions in this restricted area involve innumerable factors: muscles, tarsal plates, conjunctiva, skin, tear ducts, the medial canthal tendon, the less well defined lateral ligament, and of course primarily the bones. In addition, from the orbital frame to the eyelids, from the canthi to the lacrimal system, from the eyebrows to the fornices and eyelashes, there are crossroads of complexity, antagonism, subtlety, and uncertainty — in front of the cornea, below the cranial fossae, beside the nasoethmoidal labyrinth, and above the maxillary sinus.

Individual articles on fractures of the orbit have flourished over the past 40 years, and especially in the last 10. This has been to a large measure due to the introduction of microplates, which provide better stability than wires, and materials for bone substitution which are designed to build up the fragile bony orbital frame around the eye and its adnexae.

There have, however, been less than a dozen books on the surgery of the eyelids and orbit since the one published by J. Mustarde in 1963, and they have all dealt with multiple aspects of a larger and even more complex region. They have also in general been the product of several co-authors, whose individual chapters have overlapped in content and differed in style and approach.

Beat Hammers's book, by contrast, concentrates exclusively on orbital fractures, rather then attempting to deal exhaustively with facial traumas. Several original and interesting features features make it a unique work.

First, it is a book by a single author who avoids useless repetitions. It is based on his experiences from operating on more than 500 traumas within the last 5 years, and this means that the examination techniques and management are more homogeneous than in a practice that is spread over one or two generations. Secondly, the text is clear, concise, and does not digress. The illustrations speak for themselves, and the radiograms and CTs are just what a reader always hopes for, but rarely gets. Remarkably, almost half of the CTs are from the coronal view (except when the author wants to demonstrate exophthalmos in an axial cut), which corresponds to the angle of vision used for the clinical examination of patients and and how we observe people in real life.

Thirdly, the surgical indications are based on common sense. In the treatment of bony defects, autogenic bone grafts leave little place – if any – for the use of allogenic materials. In this regard, 50 years of experience have demonstrated that the quick-acting allogenic procedures are often disappointing in the medium term.

Fourthly, it will be noticed how scrupulous the analysis of results is, and how comprehensive the sections on complications.

And finally, the sketches and drawings have been done by Beat Hammer himself, who has found a graphical means of expression ideally suited to the orbital area.

Orbital Fractures only shows a sample of Beat Hammer's work in the department of Prof. Prein in Basel, where he practices orthognathic surgery and works on facial and craniofacial malformations. A foreword is a comment on a present work, and does not normally presume to comment on the future. However, my personal wish for the year 2000 would be for a book just as good as this, but based on even more experience, extended to include all facial traumas, and including the same quality of illustrations and graphic work.

Paul Tessier
Paris, Fall 1994

Acknowledgments

The author would like to express his gratitude to the many people who directly or indirectly contributed to this book.

First, I would like to thank Prof. Dr. J. Prein, my chairman and friend, who has been highly supportive of my clinical and scientific activities, and whose important encouragement has resulted in my preparation of this manuscipt. I would also like to thank Prof. Dr. F. Harder, Head of the Surgical Department of our hospital, for his continuous support of the project.

The most influential person responsible for stimulating my interest in orbital problems has been Dr. Paul Tessier, the "father of craniofacial surgery," who honored our unit by operating on several patients while a visiting surgeon in Basel. It was always fascinating to watch him operate; he worked like an artist, with calm and steady movements, avoiding every unnecessary manipulation.

Dr. N. Lüscher, head of the Plastic Surgery Division of our unit, provided invaluable input for the drawings as well as for the overall structure of the book.

I would also like to express my gratitude towards Drs. H.E. Killer and D. Wieser, coauthors of Chapter 4 *(Ophthalmic Aspects),* for their essential assistance. Their constant support in the ophthalmologic follow-up of patients with orbital fractures has been invaluable.

The text was proofread by Drs. Alex Greenberg, New York, and Richard Bevilaqua, Hartford (Connecticut), U.S.A. They helped provide this book with the proper grammatical structure and at the same time gave me invaluable comments on the content.

Documentation and patient follow-up was most efficiently done by Drs. R. Hofstetter, A. Huber, Ch. Kunz, Th. Räss, A. Tschanz, R. Weber and H. Schiel.

The special subject of the book necessarily requires a number of color figures, resulting in high production costs. The generous financial support by Synthes Maxillofacial, Paoli (USA), Stratec Medical, Waldenburg (Switzerland), and Mathys, Bettlach (Switzerland) enabled the completion of this project.

I would like to thank Mr. J. Flury and Mr. Robert Dimbleby of Hogrefe & Huber Publishers for their constant support and their thorough reproduction of drawings and photographs.

A final word of thanks goes to the patients, who generously allowed me to publish their photos. The book is dedicated to all of them.

Table of Contents

Chapter 1: Introduction   1

Chapter 2: Surgical Anatomy of the Orbit   2

    Definition of the Key Area   2
    The Orbital Fissures   2
    Vascularization   3
    The Orbital Connective Tissue
       System   3
    Distances and Landmarks   4
    Anatomic Basis of Posttraumatic
       Enophthalmos   5

Chapter 3: Diagnosis and Classification   7

3.1 Fracture Patterns and Their Classification   7
    Classification of Orbito-Zygomatic
       Fractures   7
    Classification of Naso-Orbito-Ethmoid
       Fractures   8
    Internal Orbital Fracture Patterns   10
    Combined Orbital Fractures   11
3.2 Associated Injuries in Orbital Fractures   12
3.3 Diagnosis   13
    Clinical Examination   13
    Plain Radiographs   13
    CT Examination   14
    Other Imaging Techniques   17

Chapter 4: Ophthalmic Aspects   18

4.1 Visual Impairment   18
    Mechanisms   18
    Diagnosis   20
    Management of Traumatic Visual Loss   21
    Visual Loss Following Fracture Repair   23
    Case Reports   23
4.2 Diplopia   24
    Mechanisms   24
    Diagnosis and Documentation   26
    Management   27

Chapter 5: Conservative Treatment   29

Chapter 6: Database   31

6.1 Review of Patients with Primary Repair   31
    Patient Population   31
    Fracture Patterns and Associated Injuries   32
    Operative Treatment   33
    Follow-Up   34
6.2 Review of Patients with Secondary
       Corrections   40
    Patient Population and Type of Deformities   40
    Operative Treatment   40
    Results   41

**Chapter 7: Operative Management of
Orbital Fractures**   43

7.1 Basic Principles   43
    Exposure   43
    Rigid Fixation   45
    Bone Graft Harvesting of the Calvarium   45
    Repositioning of Soft Tissues with
       Suspension Sutures   47
7.2 Orbito-Zygomatic Fractures (Outer Orbital
       Frame)   48
    Nonfragmented Orbito-Zygomatic
       Fractures   48
    Fragmented Orbito-Zygomatic Fractures   50
7.3 Naso-Orbito-Ethmoid Fractures (Inner
       Orbital Frame)   51
    Management of the Central Fragment   51
    Nasal Reconstruction   53
    Naso-Orbito-Ethmoid Fracture-Related
       Problems   53
    Sequence of Operative Steps in Repair of
       Naso-Orbito-Ethmoidal Fractures   53
7.4 Fractures of the Internal Orbit   54
    Linear Fractures   54
    Blow-Out Fractures   54
    Complex Orbital-Wall Defects   55

7.5 Surgical Technique for the Repair of Complex Orbital Fractures	57	Skeletal Reconstruction	76
7.6 Case Reports	59	Soft Tissue Repositioning	78
7.7 Errors in Orbital Reconstruction	71	8.4 Complications	80
Exposure	71	Ocular Complications	80
Orbital Frame	71	Infections	80
Orbital Wall Reconstruction	71	Other Complications	80
		8.5 Functional Aspects	80
		Sequence of Treatment	80

Chapter 8: Secondary Corrections   73

8.6 Case Reports   80

8.1 Principles of Corrective Surgery	73	**Chapter 9: Summary and Conclusion**	**89**
Skeletal Reconstruction	73		
Soft Tissue Rearrangement	73	**Endnotes**	**91**
Multistage Correction	74		
8.2 Diagnosis	74	**References**	**93**
8.3 Surgical Technique	74		
Exposure	74	**Subject Index**	**99**

Chapter 1
Introduction

The orbit is involved in more than 40% of all facial injuries [1], with a variety of presentations: orbito-zygomatic, naso-orbito-ethmoid, internal orbit, and combinations thereof. There is also considerable variation in the severity of injuries, ranging from simple nondisplaced to complex comminuted fractures. These complex fractures amount to about 20% of the total (see Chapter 6), though they are responsible for the majority of complications and unfavorable results.

This book provides the reader with guidelines for the identification and diagnosis of simple to severe orbital injuries, thus facilitating surgical decision making and filling the need for a description of basic or advanced (extended approach) operative techniques.

A database is included with a review of 443 patients (constituting 78% of 513 patients treated during the last 5 years) as well as 26 patients operated on for late sequelae in the same period.

Complex orbital fractures still present a challenge, even to the experienced surgeon, and a large number of problems are still to be solved. The techniques described in this book, however, have currently proved to allow predictable reconstruction of the severely injured orbit.

Chapter 2
Surgical Anatomy of the Orbit

The orbit is a complex structure, composed of seven individual bones. It has the shape of a four-sided pyramid with an open apex, the base being formed by the orbital rim. Through the open apex, nerves and vessels enter the orbit in order to allow the function of the visual organ.

Yet it is not a pure quadrilateral pyramid, but rather in cross-section quadrilateral at the base and triangular at the apex. This change in configuration towards the apex results from the blending of the posterior third of the orbital floor into the medial wall, where they merge.

It is assumed that the reader is familiar with the descriptive anatomy of the bony orbit as well as of the eye and its adnexae, excellent publications on this topic being available [9–13].

This chapter highlights some aspects of practical importance regarding the exposure and reconstruction of the traumatically injured bony orbit.

For surgical purposes, the orbit can be subdivided into two main components:
- orbital frame
- orbital walls or pyramid.

The orbital frame is a thick bony structure including the orbital rim and the zygomatic arch (Figures 2.1, 2.2). It is a part of the midface buttressing system [14].

The thin orbital walls form an open pyramid, the characteristics of which are described above. Some elements of this pyramidal system have certain implications in the repair of orbital wall fractures and will therefore be described in greater detail:
- the key area (see below for definition)
- orbital fissures
- the vascularization pattern of the orbital contents
- the orbital connective tissue system.

Definition of the Key Area

The posterior medial wall is an area of special importance in orbital reconstruction and for this reason is called the *key area*:

- The posterior medial wall, together with the posterior lateral wall, form the main support for the anterior projection of the globe by their fan-like divergence anteriorly and superiorly. The function of the two walls has been compared to a pair of cupped hands holding the globe in its forward position [15].
- Being a paper-thin structure, it is often damaged in orbital injuries.
- Clinical experience has shown that repair of fractures with an intact key area is technically much easier than repair of injuries involving this part of the orbit. Therefore, the first step in the repair of complex orbital fractures is reconstruction of the key area employing rigid fixation techniques [16], described in Section 7.4.

The Orbital Fissures

At the apex of the orbital pyramid, the superior orbital fissure opens into the middle cranial fossa, allowing the cranial nerves III, IV, V and VI to enter the orbit in a well-defined spatial relationship.

The inferior orbital fissure communicates with the retromaxillary space and is traversed by several small arteries. Posteriorly, it blends into the superior orbital fissure. The transition between the superior and interior orbital fissure is a weak spot of the orbit, because fractures of the orbital floor extending laterally and posteriorly may result in an enlargement of the fissure, allowing the orbital contents to herniate, thus leading to enophthalmos (Figure 2.3 a–

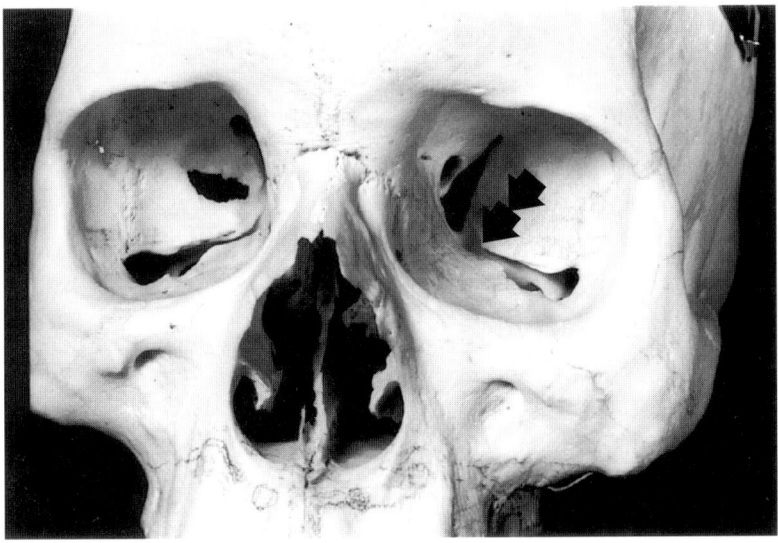

Figure 2.1. The bony orbit. Note that the cross-section of the deep cone is triangular, while it is quadrilateral in the anterior part, owing to the orbital floor blending posteriorly into the medial wall. The clinical implications of this finding are mentioned in the text.

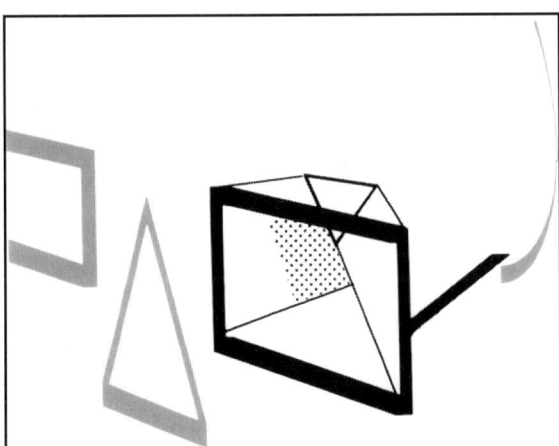

Figure 2.2. Schematic drawing of the orbit showing the two main components: orbital frame and orbital pyramid. The shaded area represents the posteromedial wall (key area).

c). Repair of these fractures should include complete obliteration of the inferior orbital fissure [17].

Vascularization

The eye and adnexae present an axial vascularization pattern originating from the ophthalmic artery which enters the orbit through the optic canal, below the optic nerve. This anatomic relationship permits safe subperiosteal dissection of the entire orbital contents back to the deep cone. Several small vessels without significant importance penetrating the orbital walls are routinely divided during dissection. In the anterior part of the lateral wall, a small zygomatico-orbital artery is encountered, and several small vessels branch into the periorbita from the infraorbital neurovascular bundle. The anterior ethmoid artery usually requires division to allow adequate exposure, while the posterior ethmoid artery (only 3–5 mm anterior to the optic canal) is preserved.

The Orbital Connective Tissue System

Between the orbital walls, the muscles and the globe there is a highly organized system of connective tissue septae that is obviously involved in normal eye movements [21] (Figure 2.4). The septae, embedded in periorbital fat, are able to slide against each other, simultaneously securing normal eye position and motility.

Disruption of the periorbit in orbital wall fractures may result in adhesions between the septae, leading to motility problems, especially in the case of inadequate fracture repair and consecutive healing of the septae in a distorted position (see Section 4.2, Figure 4.8). This seems to be the main factor in the development of restrictive motility disorder.

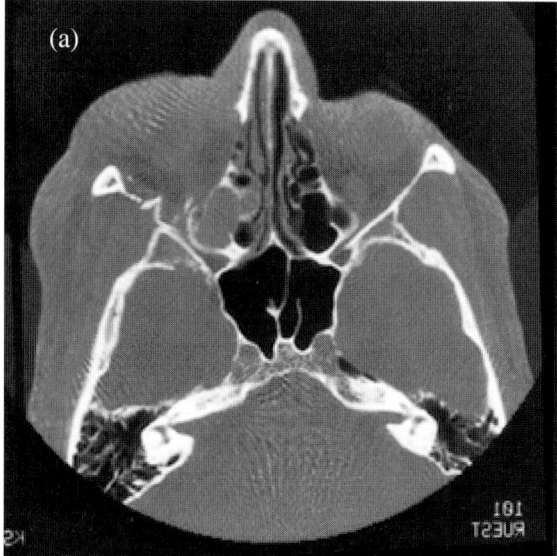

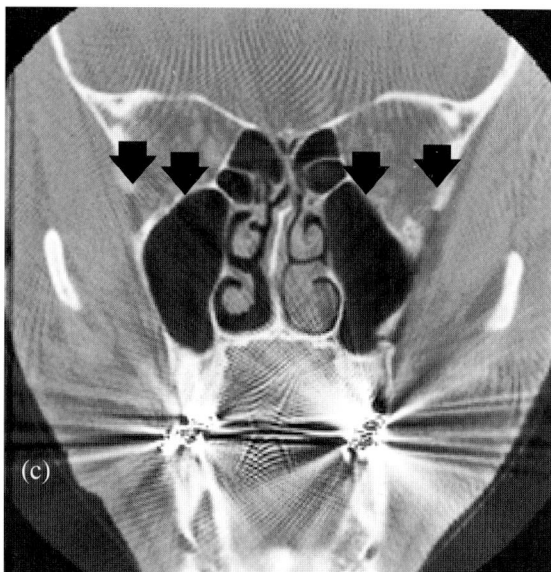

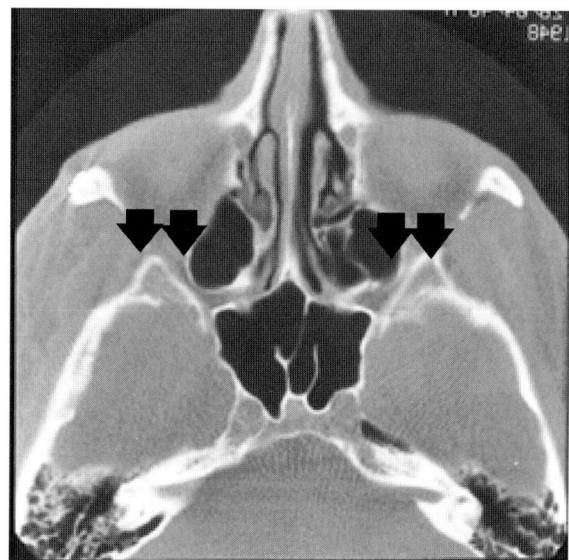

Figure 2.3 (a-c). (a) CT scan of an orbito-zygomatic fracture with an orbital floor defect extending into the infraorbital fissure (arrow). (b) and (c) Axial and coronal CT scan 1 year after the accident. A dent has formed resulting in a widening of the inferior orbital fissure (arrows). There is mild (2 mm) enophthalmos. The clinical picture of the patient is shown in Figure 6.4.

Distances and Landmarks

In order to provide data for safe dissection, gauging of the orbits has been performed on cadaveric skulls as well as on CT scans [18, 19]. In the heavily injured orbit, however, these values may become irrelevant because the landmarks themselves are dislocated. Instead of relying on so-called safe distances, one carries out dissection of the deep orbit strictly in a subperiosteal plane, allowing direct visualization of the borders of the superior orbital fissure as well as the optic canal.

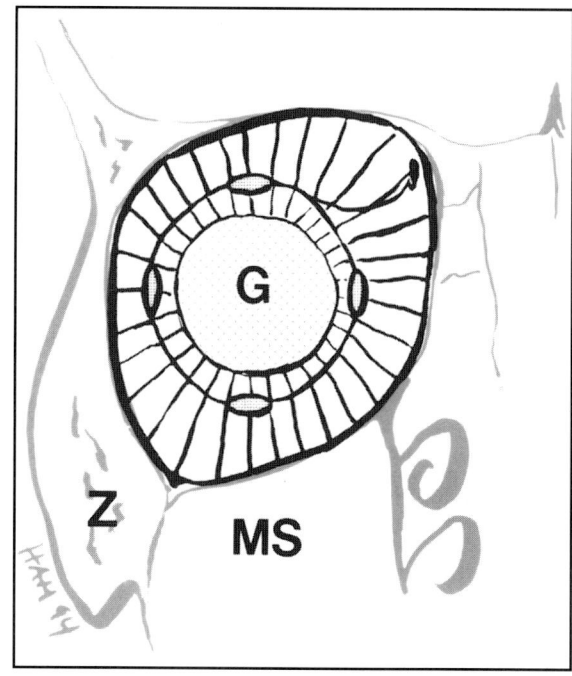

Figure 2.4. Schematic cross-section of the orbit showing the ligament system. The system consists of connective tissue lamella arranged in a 3-dimensional fashion. Their function is to hold the globe in a defined position, yet allow free mobility. G: ocular globe, Z: zygoma, MS: maxillary sinus (Redrawn after Koorneef, L. Spatial aspects of the orbital musculo-fibrous tissue in man. Amsterdam and Lisse: Swets and Zeitlinger (1977), with permission).

Gauging the orbit has also been performed to evaluate the possibility of manufacturing preshaped orbital implants for the repair of orbital wall defects [20]. The high interindividual differences and the variability of orbital shapes found in dried skulls, however, do not favor this idea. Nevertheless, orbital floor plates that can be individually shaped have found wide use in orbital fracture repair [16].

Anatomic Basis of Post-traumatic Enophthalmos

Enophthalmos is a common sequel to complex orbital fractures, and its mechanisms, prevention and correction have been widely discussed in the literature [7, 15, 22, 23, 24]. Theories on the mechanisms include enlargement of the bony orbit, fat atrophy, and scar contracture. Of all these factors, anatomic and volumetric changes of the bony orbit most significantly affect globe position [7, 24]. The aim of fracture treatment must therefore be the restoration of the preinjury shape and volume of the bony orbit.

In the primate model, defects in the posterior part of the orbit, lying b(ehind the globe axis, produce enophthalmos, while defects in the anterior part of the orbital floor do not change the antero-posterior globe position [22]. However, reconstruction of the

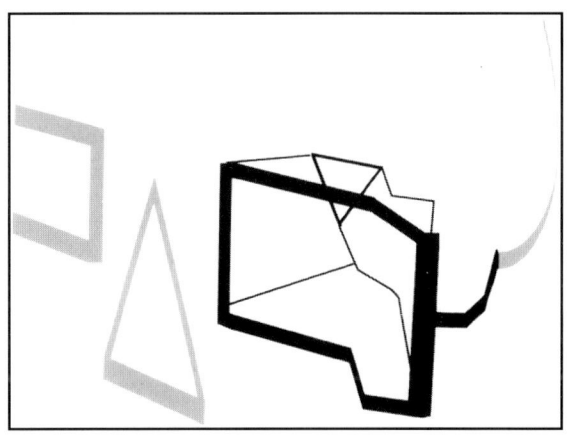

Figure 2.5. Incorrect reduction of the zygoma produces orbital enlargement by leaving a defect in the lateral wall.

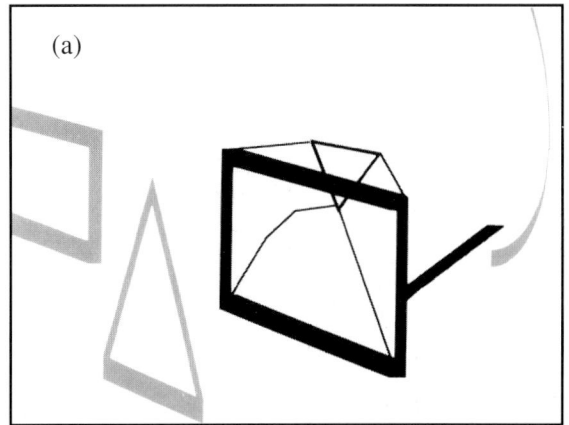

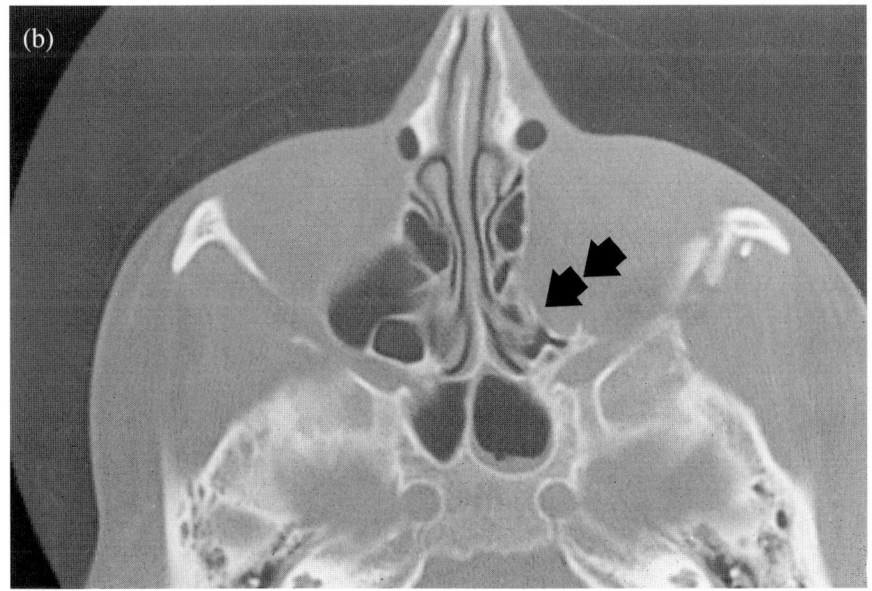

Figure 2.6 (a, b). Inadequate reconstruction of the posterior medial wall (key area) produces an enlargement of the posterior orbit, resulting in enophthalmos. Schematic drawing (a, above) and CT scan (b) of patient no. 8.4 (see Figure 8.10). Arrows in (b) indicate enlarged posterior orbit.

anterior orbital floor is necessary to maintain vertical globe position.

The two main errors producing enlargement of the postbulbar orbit are:
– incorrect reduction of zygomatico-orbital fractures, resulting in malrotation of the zygomatic body and leaving a defect in the lateral orbital wall which allows orbital contents to escape (Figure 2.5);
– inadequate reconstruction of the posterior medial wall (Figure 2.6). In our own patients, this was found to be the most important technical error in complex orbital fracture repair (see also Section 7.8).

Chapter 3
Diagnosis and Classification

3.1 Fracture Patterns and Their Classification

Fractures involving the orbit may affect a part of or the entire orbit. They are referred to as follows:
- *Orbito-zygomatic fractures* (OZM), if the malar complex is the main area of impact,
- *Naso-orbito-ethmoid fractures* (NOE), if the trauma is essentially directed to the central midface,
- *Internal orbital fractures* (blow-out, blow-in), confined to the orbital walls, and
- *Combined orbital fractures*, involving major parts or the entire orbital skeleton.

Classification of Orbito-Zygomatic Fractures

Orbito-zygomatic fractures are the most common injuries involving the orbit and in fact are the most frequently encountered facial fractures [1]. They exhibit considerable variations in their degrees of severity, ranging from nondisplaced nonfragmented fractures to highly fragmented injuries.

A variety of classifications has been proposed [25–28], the majority of them describing four basic fracture patterns (Figure 3.1):

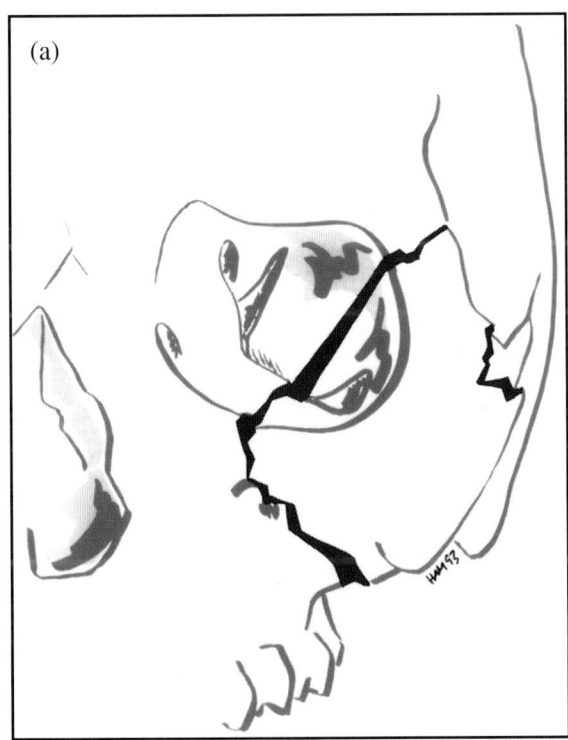
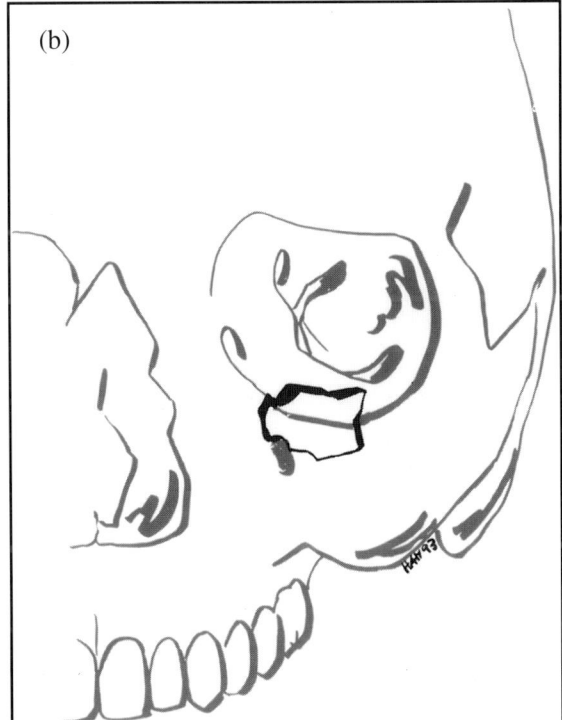

Figure 3.1 (a, b). Orbito-zygomatic (OZM) fracture patterns. (a) Orbito-zygomatic fracture Type I: Nondisplaced or minimally displaced OZM fracture. Closed reduction is usually sufficient. (b) Orbito-zygomatic fracture Type II: Segmental fracture of the infraorbital rim. Open reduction and stabilization with microplates is necessary to restore the continuity of the infraorbital rim.

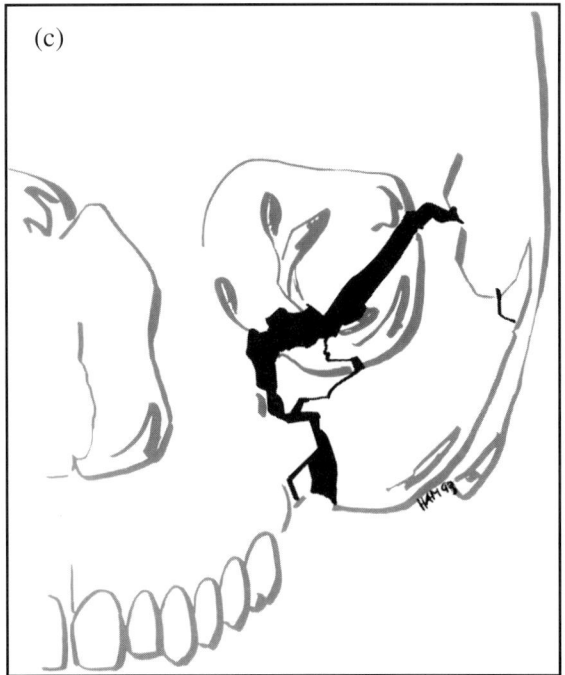
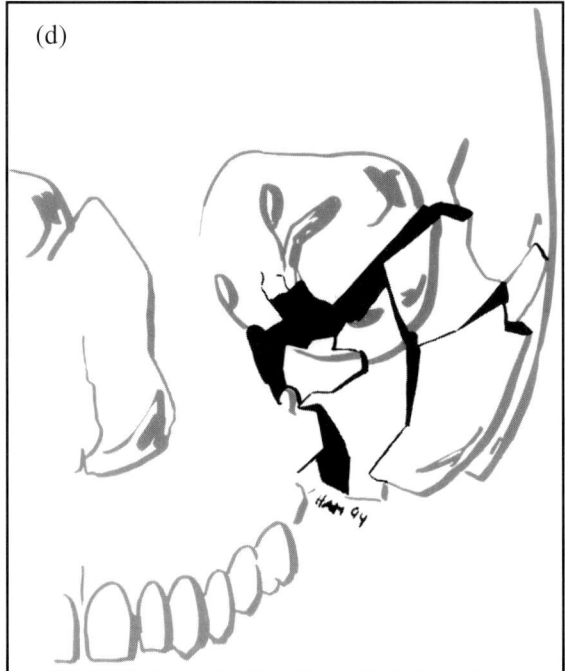

Figure 3.1 (c, d). (c) Orbito-zygomatic fracture Type III: The zygomatic body is fractured en bloc. There is, however, an isolated fragment at the infraorbital rim and often at the zygomatico-maxillary buttress as well. Open reduction and internal fixation is necessary to avoid secondary dislocation. These fractures are often associated with a small anterior defect in the orbital floor (blow-out type). (d) Orbito-zygomatic fracture Type IV: Fragmented orbito-zygomatic fracture. These fractures result from high-velocity injuries and are usually associated with defects of the orbital walls. Correct three-dimensional reconstruction requires an extended approach.

- segmental fractures,
- nondisplaced or minimally displaced nonfragmented fractures of the zygoma,
- displaced fractures of the zygomatic body, usually with an isolated fragment at the inferior orbital rim and/or at the zygomatico-maxillary buttress, and
- fragmented orbito-zygomatic fractures.

The classification proposed by Jackson [25] (Table 3.1) classifies the severity of the fracture, *not* the direction of displacement, and thus indicates the importance of a pattern-related surgical approach.

Table 3.1. Classification of orbito-zygomatic fractures (after Jackson).

Fracture type	Severity of injury	Type of trauma
Type I	nondisplaced	low velocity
Type II	segmental	localized
Type III	tripod	low velocity
Type IV	fragmented*	high velocity

*Type IV orbito-zygomatic fractures are typically associated with orbital wall defects extending posteriorly into the key area.

Jackson clearly identifies the fragmented orbito-zygomatic fracture as an injury requiring extensive exposure and stabilization.

Classification of Naso-Orbito-Ethmoid Fractures

The naso-orbito-ethmoid area exhibits a complex three-dimensional anatomy, the integrity of which is essential for facial esthetics. Blunt trauma to the central midface produces fractures occurring along the lines of least resistance. The displacement of fragments results in a flattening of the nose combined with increased intercanthal distance.

Although there is a considerable variation in the fracture patterns occurring either uni- or bilaterally, three basic types of injury can be distinguished, essentially differing in the size of the "central," canthal ligament-bearing fragment produced by the impact [29] (Figure 3.2):

- Type I injuries exhibit a large central fragment consisting of the entire medial portion of the or-

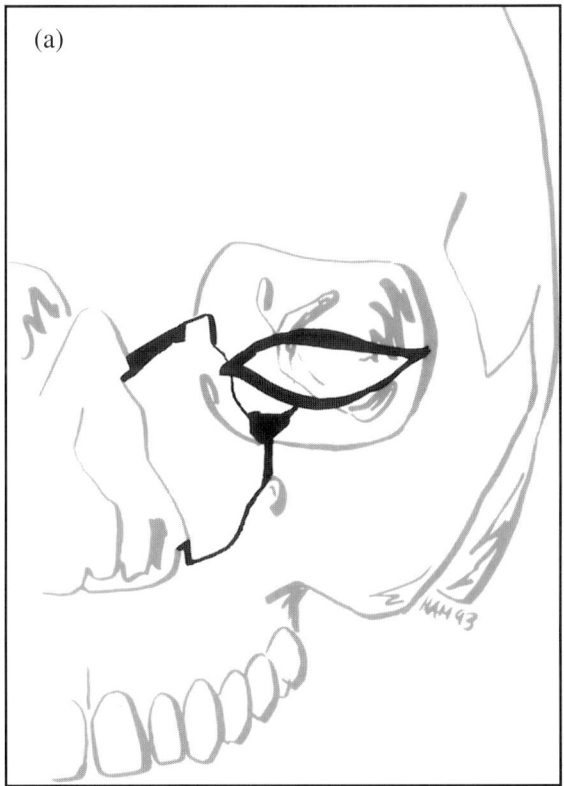
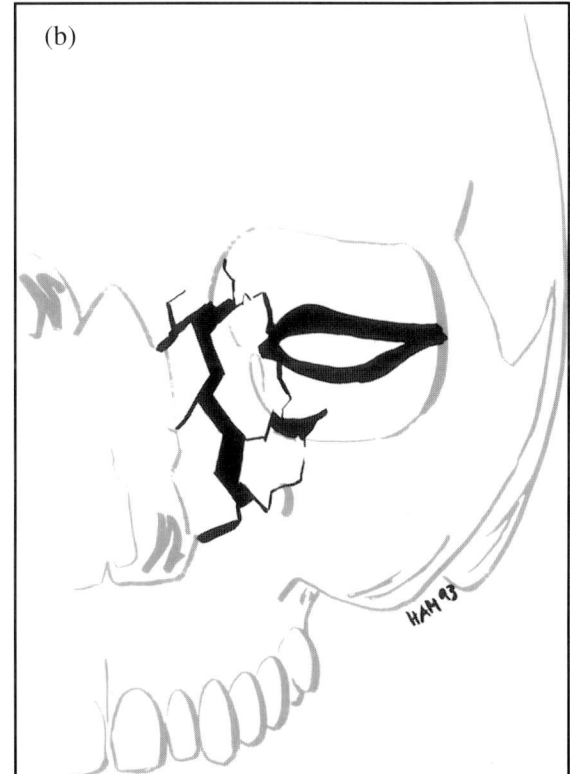
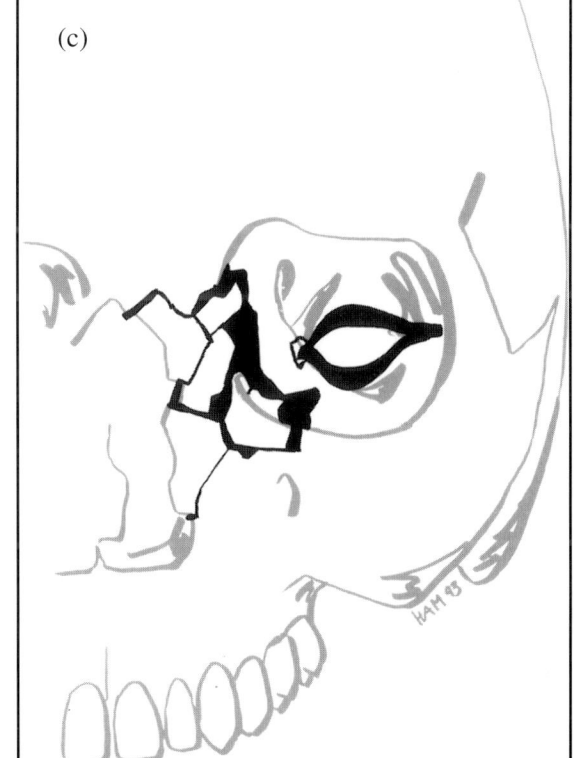

Figure 3.2 (a-c). Naso-orbito-etmoid (NOE) fracture patterns. (a) Naso-orbito-ethmoid fracture Type I: There is one large central fragment. Correct three-dimensional reduction and fixation anatomically restores the canthal area. (b) Naso-orbito-ethmoid fracture Type II: There is some degree of fragmentation, but the ligament-bearing fragment is large enough to be grasped and stabilized. (c) Naso-orbito-ethmoid fracture Type III: There is only a small canthal-ligament-bearing fragment or complete avulsion of the ligament has occurred. Direct transnasal canthopexy is necessary.

bital rim (inner facial frame), with the ligament attached to the lacrimal crest.
– Type II injuries exhibit disruption of the inner frame into several fragments, with the ligament-bearing fragment being sufficiently large to undergo fixation.
– Type III injuries exhibit a high degree of comminution of the central fragment. The canthal ligament-bearing segment is only a few millimeters large and therefore cannot be stabilized surgically. In rare instances there may be complete avulsion of the ligament.

Adequate reestablishment of the preinjury intercanthal distance as well as of the correct position of the ligament posterior to the lacrimal crest (perhaps even more important) is the key to successful manage-

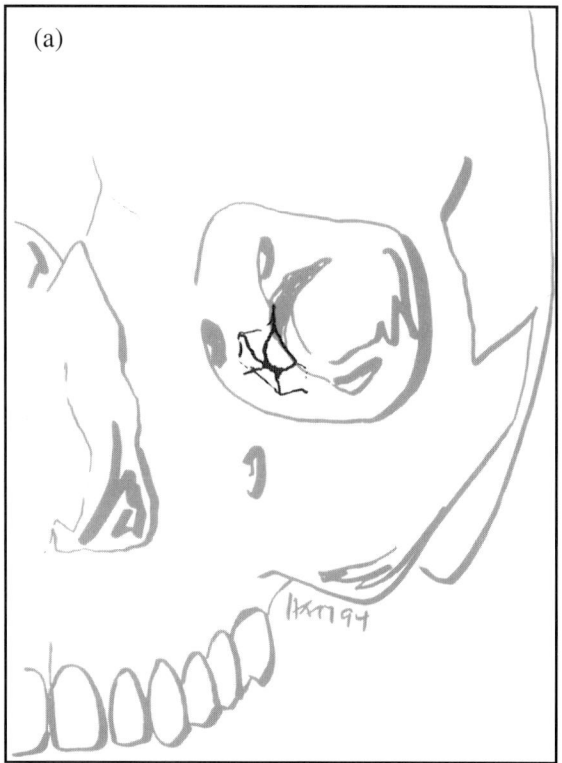
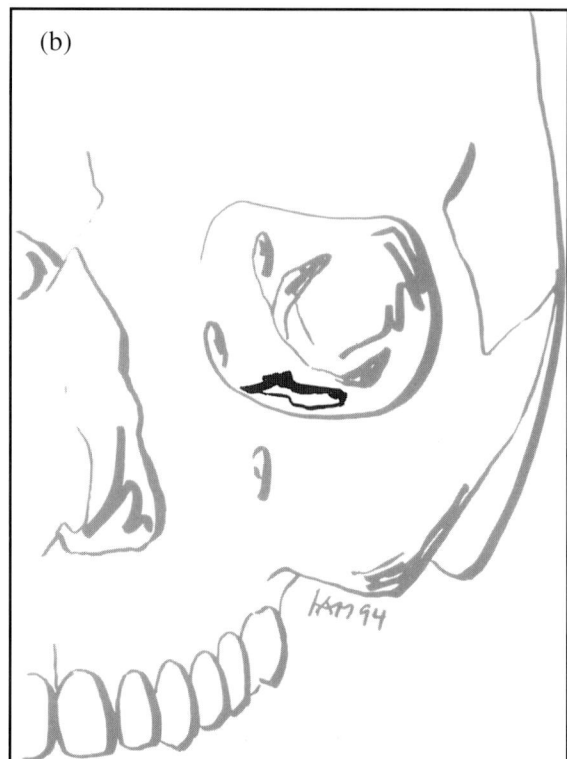
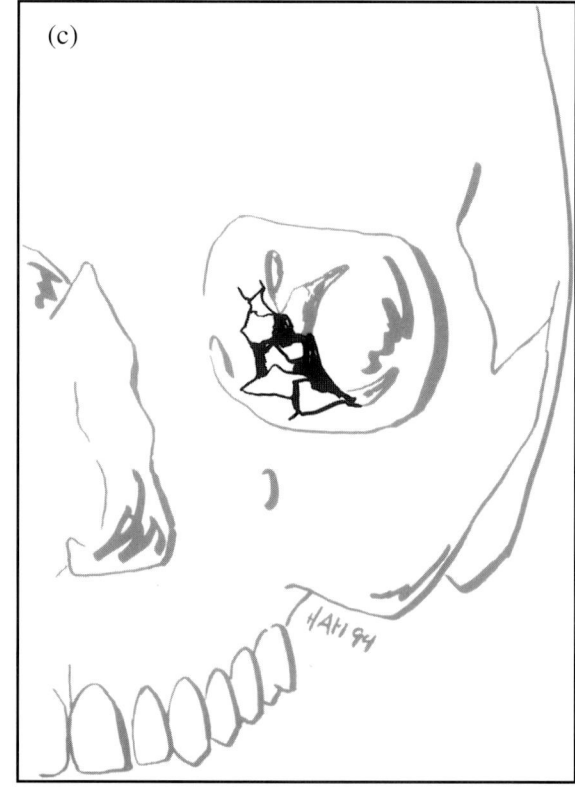

Figure 3.3 (a-c). Fractures of the internal orbit. (a) Linear fracture: Minor trauma or trauma not primarily directed to the orbital floor may produce an eggshell type of orbital wall fracture, without defect. If no repair is performed, localized enlargement of the orbit occurs. (b) Blow-out or blow-in fracture: These fractures are confined to one wall, usually the orbital floor (see also Figure 3.4). (c) Complex fracture of the internal orbit: Defects involving more than one wall and extending back into the orbital cone are difficult to repair because there is little or no posterior support for grafts. Complex orbital wall defects are usually associated with fractures of the orbital frame.

ment of these fractures. Pattern-based techniques for the stabilization of the central fragment are described in Chapter 7.

Internal Orbital Fracture Patterns

To our knowledge, no classification of internal orbital fractures exists to date. Parameters characterizing these fractures include the type and size as well as localization and extension of the defect into the postero-medial wall (key area). We have observed the following patterns of injuries (Figure 3.3):
– *Linear fractures.* This type of injury may be compared to the fracture of an eggshell, with the frag-

ments still being attached one to another. Although there is no real defect, significant enlargement of the orbit may occur, resulting in enophthalmos if no repair is undertaken.
- *Blow-out fractures:* The most commonly occurring injury to the orbital walls is a defect of up to 2 cm in diameter, limited to one wall. These defects are usually localized in the anterior or middle part of the orbital floor, and are referred to as blow-out fractures in accordance with their hypothetical pathological mechanism[1]. However, isolated single wall fractures are also observed in the medial orbital wall, as well as in the orbital roof, where they often present as blow-in fractures [33].
- *Complex fractures of the internal orbit:* High velocity trauma produces defects affecting two, three, or all four walls of the orbit. These defects extend back into the deep orbital cone and may even involve the optic canal. Their complex shape as well as loss of posterior support for grafts makes reconstruction a highly difficult task. Complex orbital wall defects are usually associated with fractures of the inner and/or outer orbital frame. However, isolated two-wall defects extending into the key area may be observed and should not be underestimated.

Combined Orbital Fractures

High-velocity injuries result in major disruptions of the orbital skeleton. These fractures affect the main parts of the orbital frame and several orbital walls, in most cases involving the key area (Figure 3.5). Early operative management using craniofacial techniques is mandatory to avoid severe functional and esthetic sequelae.

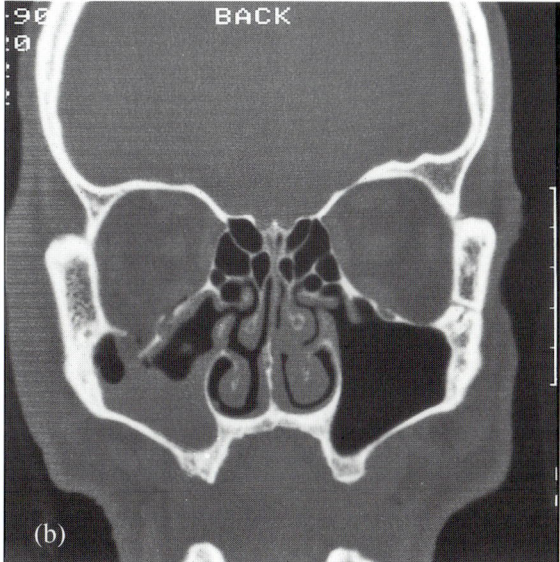

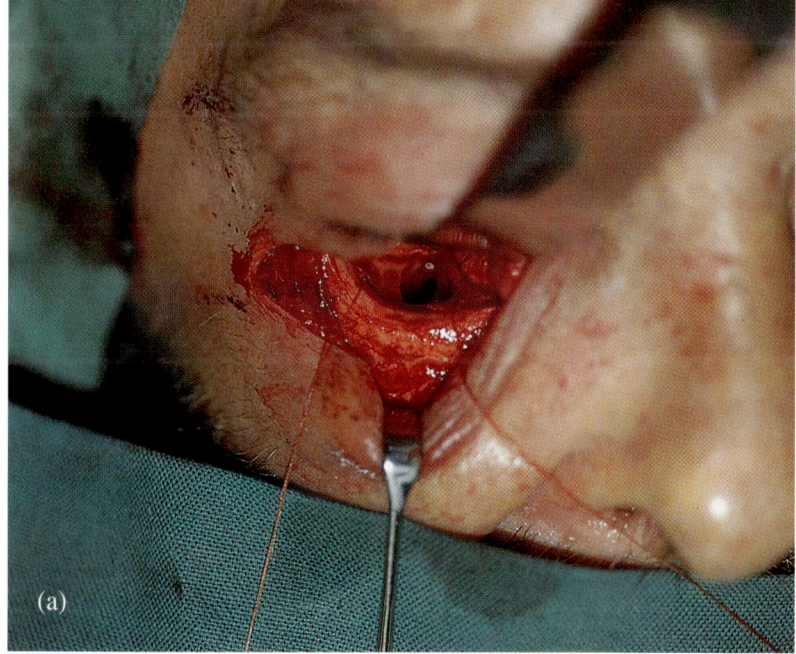

Figure 3.4 (a, b). Intraoperative view (a, left) and coronal CT scan (b, above) of a blow-out fracture involving the orbital floor.

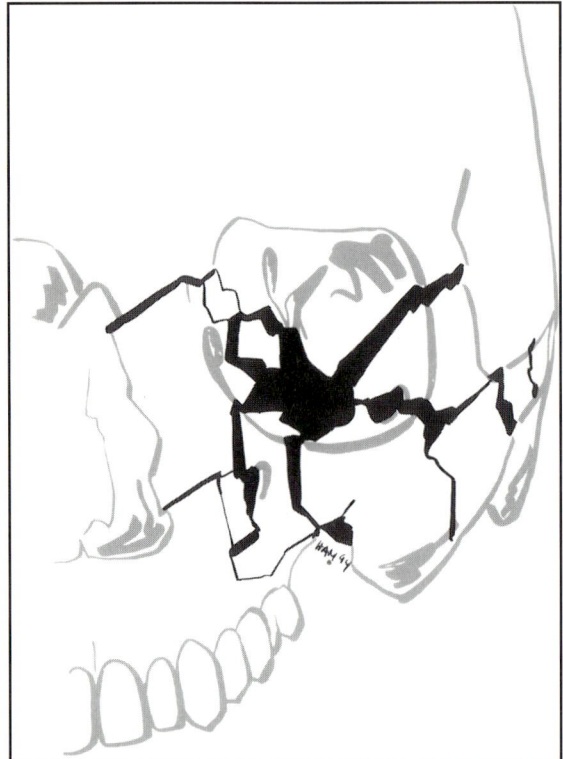

Figure 3.5. Combined orbital fracture involving the entire orbital skeleton. For repair, an extended approach with the use of craniofacial techniques is required.

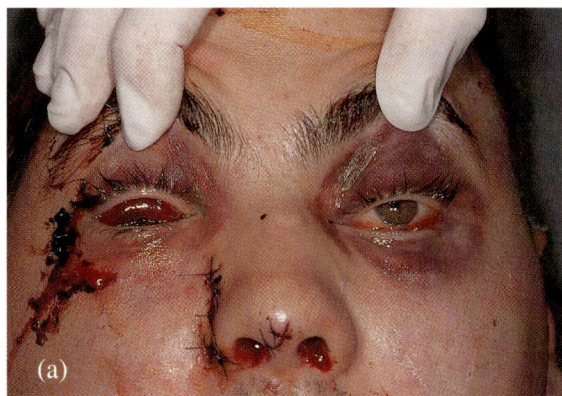

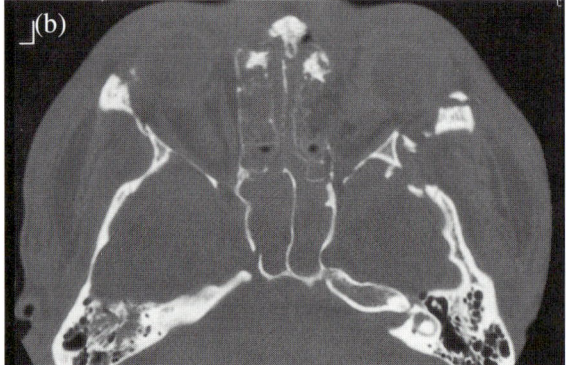

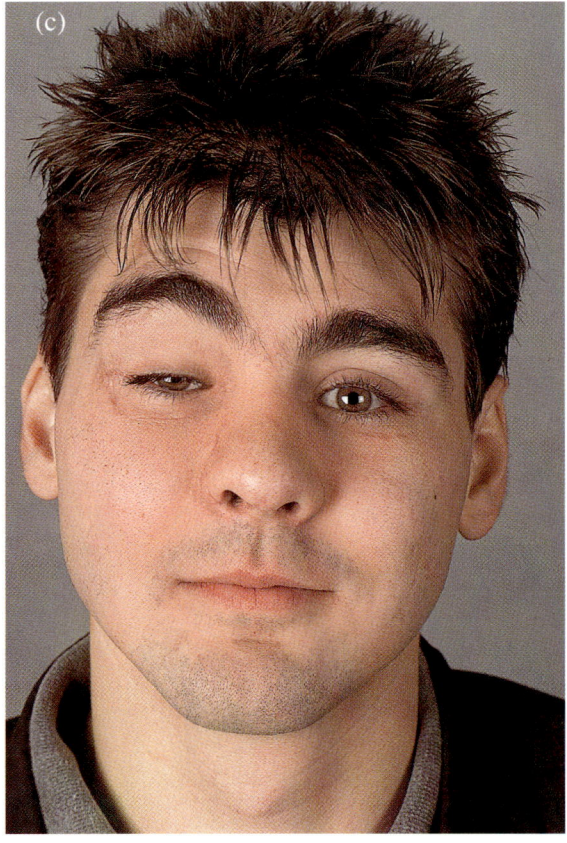

Figure 3.6 (a-c). Superior orbital fissure syndrome. (a) + (b) A combined fracture of the right orbit involving the greater sphenoid wing, resulting in a superior orbital fissure syndrome. (c) The patient 6 months after the injury, with residual ptosis of the upper lid. Botulinum toxin injections have been employed in the treatment of his 6th nerve palsy (see Chapter 4.2), allowing for binocular vision if the head is tilted slightly.

3.2 Associated Injuries in Orbital Fractures

Trauma to the bony orbit frequently affects related and neighboring structures. Typical problems associated with orbital fractures are:
- Injuries to the eye and adnexae, potentially resulting in serious impairment of visual function. Early detection and adequate treatment is of utmost importance (see Chapter 4).
- The superior orbital fissure syndrome/orbital apex syndrome: Hematoma in the posterior orbit or a dislocated fracture of the greater sphenoid wing (Figure 3.6) may result in compression of the su-

perior orbital fissure with dysfunction of cranial nerves III, IV, V and VI. Clinical symptoms of the superior orbital fissure syndrome are retrobulbar pain, internal ophthalmoplegia, upper lid ptosis and sensory disturbance of cranial nerve V_1 [34, 35]. There is usually a spontaneous, though often incomplete, recovery [36]. The combination of superior orbital fissure syndrome with optic nerve involvement is referred to as orbital apex syndrome [35, 37].
– Naso-orbito-ethmoid fractures are frequently associated with frontal sinus and skull base injuries (see Section 7.3).

3.3 Diagnosis

Clinical Examination

The clinical picture of orbital fractures is rather uniform, and for the inexperienced examiner it may be difficult to detect the discrete clinical signs indicating the presence of a complex injury. Meticulous clinical examination is of utmost importance in order to decide on further diagnostic and therapeutic procedures, by
– Providing an overview over the extent and localization of orbital and facial injuries.
– Identifying associated ocular injuries requiring ophthalmologic consultation. An algorithm for rapid clinical assessment of the eyes and adnexae (rapid ophthalmologic assessment, ROA) is described in Chapter 4.
– Identifying patients requiring CT examination of the orbits. Although clinical examination of the internal orbit is not possible, clinical and ophthalmological signs pointing toward serious trauma to the internal orbit do exist. These signs include enophthalmos, vertical globe malposition and exophthalmos. Enophthalmos and vertical globe malposition immediately after trauma indicate serious disruption of the internal orbit and therefore mandate CT scans. Severe exophthalmos, especially when associated with retrobulbar pain and decreased visual acuity, is highly indicative of retrobulbar hematoma and requires urgent CT examination and decompressive surgery when indicated (see also Section 4.1). Motility disorders and double vision are common findings immediately after trauma and may be due to edema.

However, limitations of gaze in one specific direction may indicate a mechanical limitation owing to soft tissue impingement or a motor nerve injury. If double vision does not improve rapidly after 48–72 hours, CT examination is indicated (motility disorders are discussed in Section 4.2).

The course of the clinical examination depends on the actual status of the patient. In an alert, oriented, and cooperative patient, the anamnestic investigation together with subjective ophthalmic tests including visual acuity and double vision reveal most of the necessary clinical information, whereas in the unconscious patient digital examination assessing steps, defects, and mobility is the most important diagnostic tool. Of specific importance is the bimanual palpation of the lacrimal crest, which is highly reliable in the assessment of instability [38].

Plain Radiographs

The projections used for the diagnosis of orbital fractures are the waters view (Figure 3.7) and the submental-vertex view.

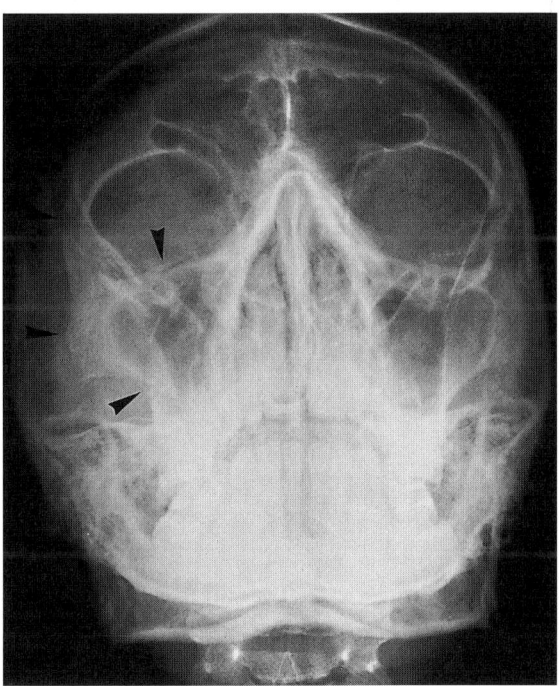

Figure 3.7. Plain-film examination of orbital fractures. The waters view projection permits detection of fractures of the zygomatic body (outer orbital frame) and in certain instances of the lacrimal crest (inner orbital frame). Fractures of the internal orbit cannot be detected directly.

Plain films can be rapidly obtained and are relatively cost-effective compared to CT scans. They allow sufficiently accurate assessment of most orbito-zygomatic fractures (outer orbital frame), but are inadequate regarding fractures of the internal orbit.

If the radiologic examination is based on plain films only, clinical signs suggestive of internal orbital fractures must be carefully considered.

The quality of standard films taken from intubated patients is mostly poor, so that CT examination is recommended on a routine basis in these situations.

Plain films are routinely obtained in the postoperative period to check the plate positions as well as the repneumatization of the paranasal sinuses.

CT Examination

CT examination is the cornerstone of orbital fracture diagnosis, permitting an exact and reproducible visualization of every part of the bony orbit as well as the adjacent structures in several planes. The diagnosis of injury to the orbital frame and orbital walls, optic canal, and skull base, as well as the paranasal sinuses and the middle and anterior cranial fossa (both of them often being involved in orbital trauma) is then radiologically possible.

The soft-tissue window enables the diagnosis of retrobulbar hematoma, optic-nerve-sheath enlargement as well as adhesions between orbital septae, eye muscles, and orbital walls.

Moreover, reproducible CT-based volumetric measurments of orbital compartments can be performed for scientific purposes [39].

This section discusses the evaluation of the bony orbit using CT scans. Typical findings related to the orbital soft tissues are described in Chapter 4 (ophthalmic aspects).

CT mandatory in the case of:
– Enophthalmos or vertical globe malposition
– Severe exophthalmos
– Retrobulbar pain
– Severe motility disorder
– Visual impairment
– Gross dislocation and/or mobility of the orbital frame

Diagnosis can best be made using high-resolution CT scans in axial and coronal planes, with a slice thickness of 2 mm. In the emergency situation, however, native coronal scans are often not obtainable because they require retroinclination of the head, which is not possible in polytraumatized patients. In uncooperative patients, image quality may further be compromised by motion artifacts, and in certain instances a delay of the CT examination by 24 to 48 hours is advisable. The benefit of optimal diagnosis, however, must be weighed against the need for immediate surgery; therefore, CT scans should be performed in severe fractures as soon as the status of the patient allows it. In virtually all cases, axial scans of average quality provide identification of the injured parts of the orbit and allow one to decide whether a limited or an extended approach to the repair is necessary (Figure 3.8).

Remarks concerning interpretation of CT scans:
– Fragmentation of the outer orbital frame is easily diagnosed on CT scans. They are especially helpful in detecting shearing fractures at the root of the zygomatic arch, requiring exposure and fixation in order to prevent shortening (see Case 7.1, Chapter 7).
– Defects of the orbital walls appear smaller on CT scans than they are in reality. The findings of Ilankovan [40] confirm our own experience.
– The presence or absence of a posterior bony ledge (Figure 3.9) is an important parameter indicating the severity of the fracture. Absence of a posterior bony ledge requires use of rigid fixation techniques for the internal orbit (see Section 6.4).
– In many cases, a defect of the orbital floor is combined with a depression of the medial wall. These fractures should not be misdiagnosed as isolated orbital floor fractures (Figure 3.10).
– The significance of a widened infraorbital fissure has been discussed in Chapter 2.
– Naso-orbito-ethmoid fractures may or may not be visible on CT scans. The bimanual examination reveals mobility, which in itself is an indication of open reduction. The degree of fragmentation often cannot be assessed preoperatively.
– 3D reformatted CT scans cannot replace axial slices in the diagnosis of orbital wall fractures. In fact, they do not add real diagnostic information and are therefore not considered to be essential.

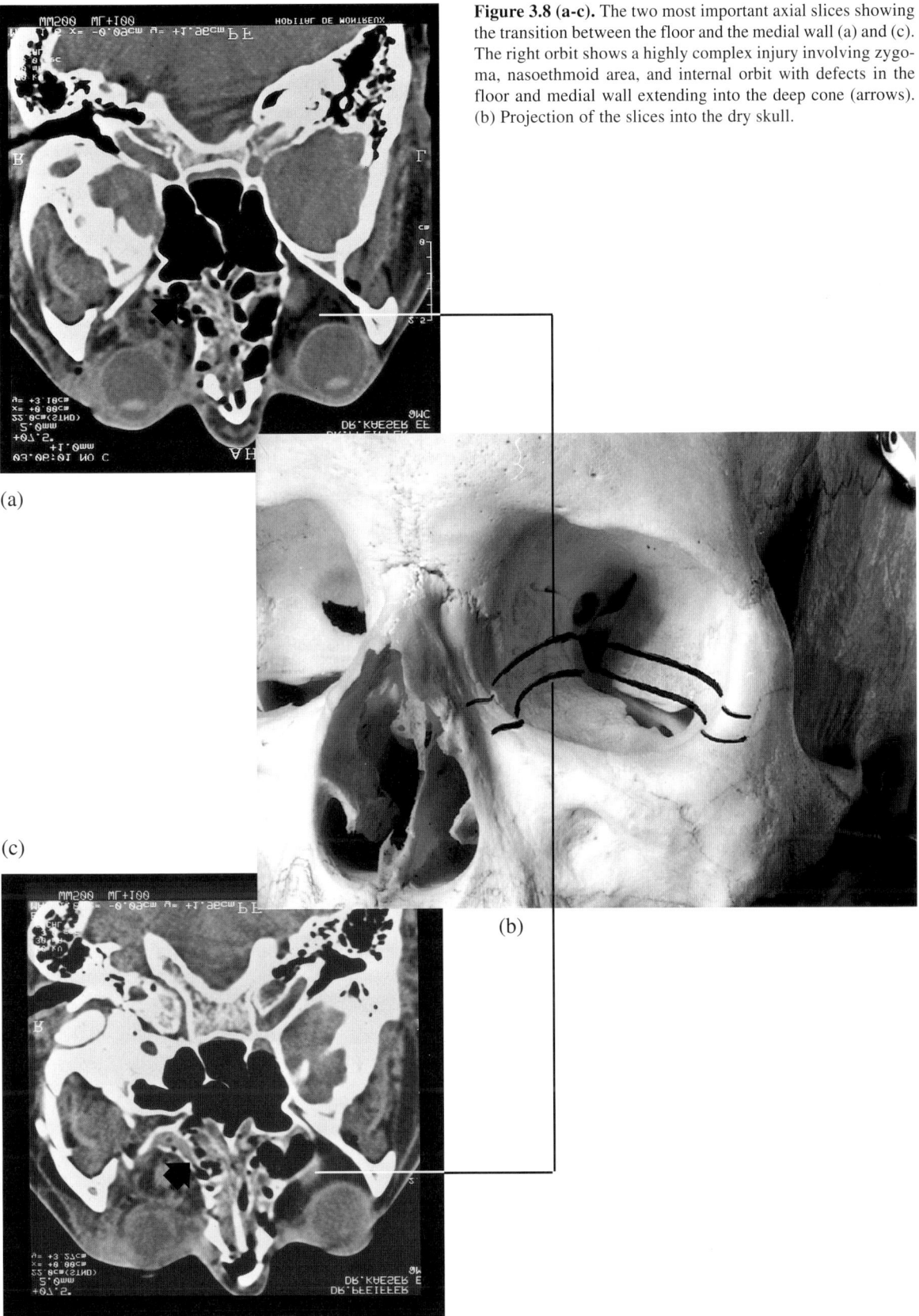

Figure 3.8 (a-c). The two most important axial slices showing the transition between the floor and the medial wall (a) and (c). The right orbit shows a highly complex injury involving zygoma, nasoethmoid area, and internal orbit with defects in the floor and medial wall extending into the deep cone (arrows). (b) Projection of the slices into the dry skull.

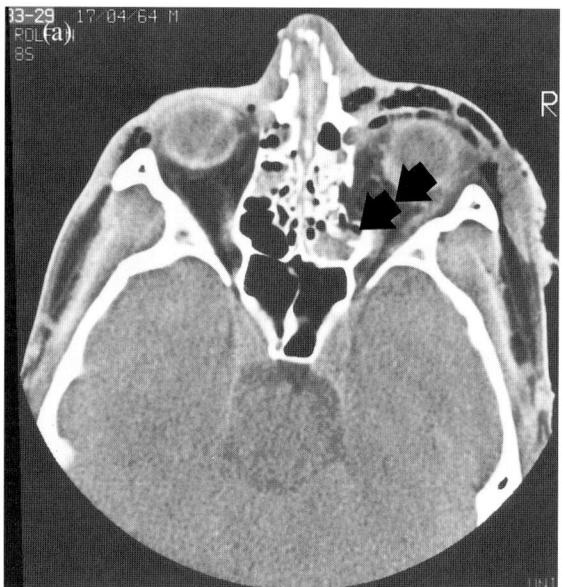
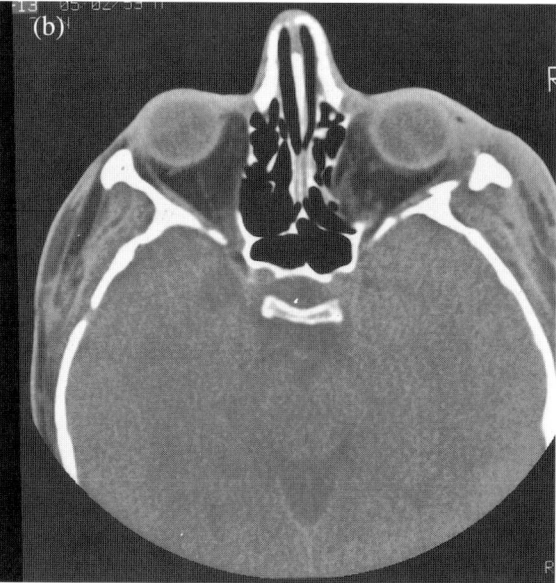

Figure 3.9 (a,b). Posterior extension of orbital wall defects. (a) A fracture involving both the right orbital floor and medial wall. However, a small posterior bony ledge (arrow) can be identified, providing support for bone grafts (coronal scan of the same patient is shown in Figure 3.10). (b) A fracture with a defect extending into the deep right orbital cone. No posterior bony ledge is identifiable, so that rigid fixation techniques are necessary (see Chapter 7).

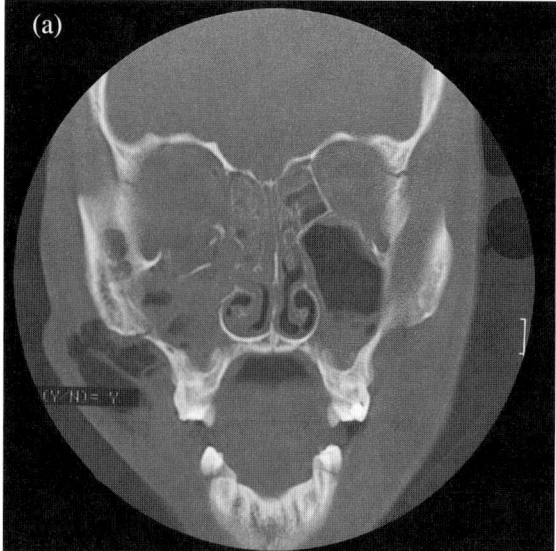
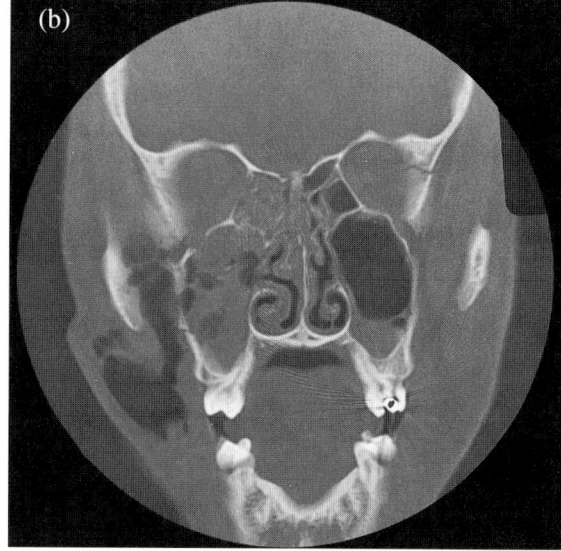

Figure 3.10. Coronal scan of the fracture shown in Figure 3.9 a. (a) The coronal scan of the middle third of the orbit shows a defect of the floor and medial wall. This is a complex fracture requiring an extended approach. (b) In the posterior part, a bony ledge can be identified, providing support for bone grafts.

Other Imaging Techniques

Apart from CT examination, other imaging techniques have been described for the diagnosis of orbital fractures. In our unit, these techniques are presently not routinely used.

Magnetic resonance imaging (MRI) has been found to be slightly superior to CT in the diagnosis of soft tissue herniation [40]; it has the additional advantage of not loading the patient with radiation. A disadvantage of present MRI examinations is the poor visibility of bony structures.

Ultrasound is a quick and noninvasive diagnostic method that has been found to be effective in the diagnosis of orbital wall defects [41], its sensitivity being comparable to that of CT imaging. However, an experienced examiner is necessary, and the defects are not as illustratively visible as on CT scans.

Solid modelling has been proposed to construct preshaped implants for orbital-wall defects [42], but we are not convinced of its practical applications in acute trauma.

Chapter 4
Ophthalmic Aspects

B. Hammer, H.E. Killer[2] and D. Wieser[3]

With orbital fractures, the two most significant effects on visual function are visual impairment or loss of visual acuity, and motility disorders, usually presenting with double vision.

4.1 Visual Impairment

Visual loss occurs in severe trauma, though minor orbital fractures and even blunt forehead trauma without loss of consciousness may also be complicated by loss of vision [43].

Initial transient decrease of visual acuity is most often due to edema of the cornea and disturbance caused by excessive lacrimation. It is important to distinguish between these conditions and serious injuries requiring immediate treatment.

Between 0.6% [44] and 14% [45] of patients with orbital fractures are reported to suffer from amaurosis or loss of vision in one eye. The incidence in our own patients was 4% [46] (Table 6.1.4).

Mechanisms

Visual impairment is caused by various traumatic mechanisms and may occur at different levels of the optic pathway (Figure 4.1).
- *Injury to the globe:* Direct or indirect trauma may result in rupture of the globe, hyphema, damage to the lens as well as vitreous hemorrhage and retinal detachment. Injuries to the anterior segment of the eye can become complicated in their course by the development of traumatic glaucoma.
- *Retrobulbar hematoma:* Visual loss due to retrobulbar hematoma (Figure 4.2) is reported by several authors [47–50], the mechanism being compression of the optic nerve by elevated intraorbital pressure. Elevated intraorbital pressure may also result from decreased orbital volume caused by severe blow-in fractures [33, 51]. Visual loss associated with elevated intraorbital pressure is an indication for immediate decompressive surgery (see below).
- *Optic nerve injury:* Damage to the optic nerve may result in a mild decrease of visual function

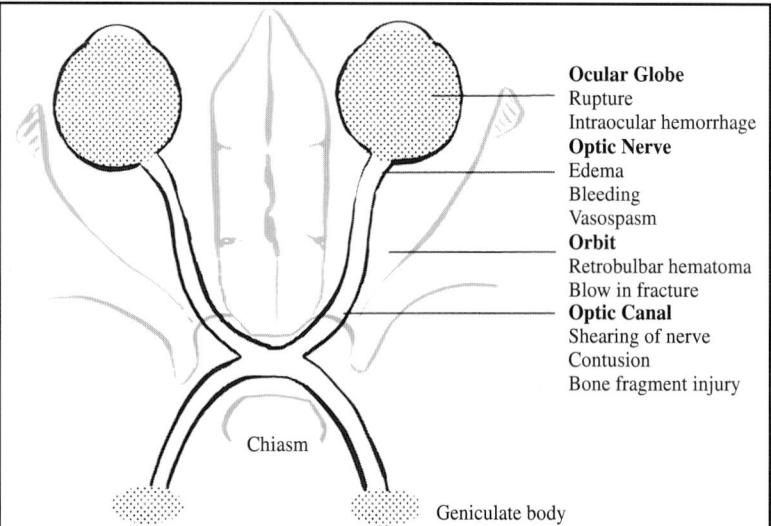

Figure 4.1. Visual function impairment may have its origin at different levels of the optic pathway (see text for details).

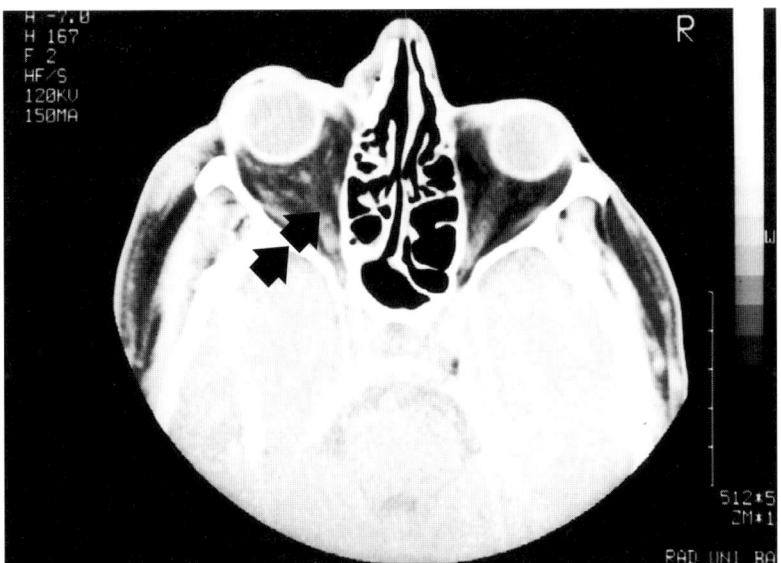

Figure 4.2. Retrobulbar hematoma of the left orbit (Case 4.1). The CT scan shows multiple hemorrhages into the retrobulbar cone (arrows).

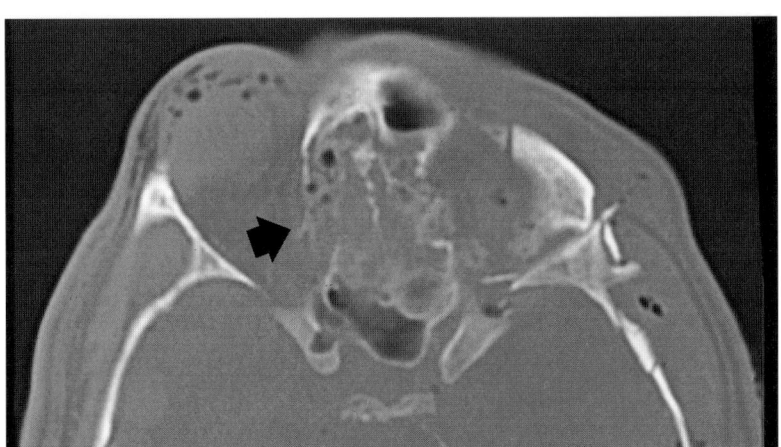

Figure 4.3. Severe blow-in fracture of the left orbit (Case 4.2): bilateral orbital fracture. A large fragment of the left medial orbital wall is displaced into the orbit (arrow). Normal vision on admission deteriorated to no light perception within 2 hours.

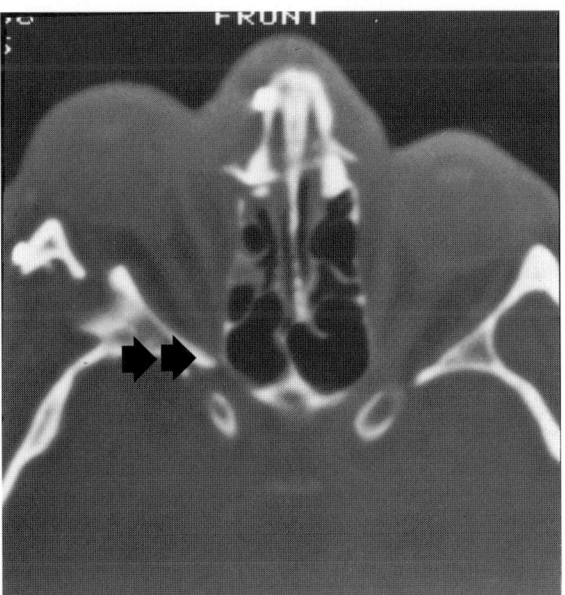

Figure 4.4. Displaced fracture of the sphenoid body, with the fragment directly transsecting the optic nerve (arrows), causing amaurosis.

to complete visual loss. The hallmarks of optic-nerve injury are decreased visual acuity, diminished color vision, and a relative afferent pupillary defect (RAPD) in the absence of globe injury. The mechanism of action may be direct or indirect (microvascular trauma).

Direct optic nerve injury occurs most likely within the optic canal, with or without fracture of the canal, the mechanism being compression, contusion, or transsection of the optic nerve along its intracanalicular pathway.

Impingement of bone fragments may cause direct transsection of the nerve (Figure 4.4), while dislocation of the optic canal may lead to disruption of the nerve by shearing forces, owing to the intimate adherence of the meninges to the periosteum in this area [52]. Primary blindness associated with bone injury in the optic canal carries a poor prognosis for visual recovery.

Indirect optic nerve injury stems from acceleration/deceleration trauma to the nerve. This type of injury leads to damage of small blood vessels with subsequent exudate followed by hypooxygenation of nerve fibres with impaired cytoplasmatic flow [53].

– *Cortical blindness:* Traumatic visual loss can also arise from contusion of the optic tract or the visual cortex, for example, in bilateral occipital contusion (the typical contre-coup injury).

Diagnosis

Patients with severe orbital fractures are often unconscious or otherwise unable to cooperate adequately. Swelling of the eyelids and chemosis further complicate the examination. While laceration of the globe is easily detected, other types of vision-threatening injuries to the eye or to the optic pathways must be thoroughly investigated.

In polytrauma patients, associated problems (bleeding, shock) may require immediate surgical intervention. A screening ophthalmologic examination must therefore take place rapidly and is thus often performed by physicians without special ophthalmologic training.

Visual acuity can deteriorate after a lucid interval, due to delayed hemorrhage, which may even occur several days after the trauma [47], making continuous monitoring of visual function mandatory. This is especially true in the unconscious patient, who is unable to complain of decreased vision.

Rapid Ophthalmologic Assessment (ROA)

Every patient with an orbital fracture should undergo a rapid screening examination to detect ophthalmological problems requiring further diagnosis or therapy. This assessment takes no more than a few minutes and can be performed without any specialized ophthalmic equipment. It includes inspection of the eye and adnexae as well as testing basic visual functions.

Rapid ophthalmologic assessment (ROA)
– Inspection (red eye, lacerations)
– Visual acuity testing
– Red and brightness saturation
– Pupillary functions (RAPD)
– Testing for double vision

Inspection
Inspection of the outer eye usually reveals gross injury to the globe. Lacerations of the eyelids always point toward globe rupture.

A red eye is a common finding, resulting most often from subconjunctival hemorrhage; this requires no therapy. Yet it may also be a sign of globe rupture or anterior chamber bleeding.

Visual Acuity Testing
Visual acuity is the basic parameter of visual assessment, though it requires a cooperative patient. The diagnosis should be as precise as the situation allows. Preprinted visual acuity charts are ideal, if available. If not, any package label may be suitable. The test object should be affixed to the patient's chart to allow later reevaluation. If applicable, the patient should wear prescription glasses for visual acuity testing.

If the patient is unable to read printed material, the maximum distance for counting fingers is recorded, or at least the ability to percieve light.

Slightly decreased visual acuity due to corneal edema and excessive tearing is common. Interpretation of visual acuity assessment must take other examinations into account, especially testing of pupillary reactions, and must be done repeatedly in order to detect any deterioration.

Red and Brightness Saturation
Red and brightness saturation is a sensitive parameter in the assessment of visual impairment. It can be tested with a flashlight, asking the patient whether there is a difference in brightness when the right or

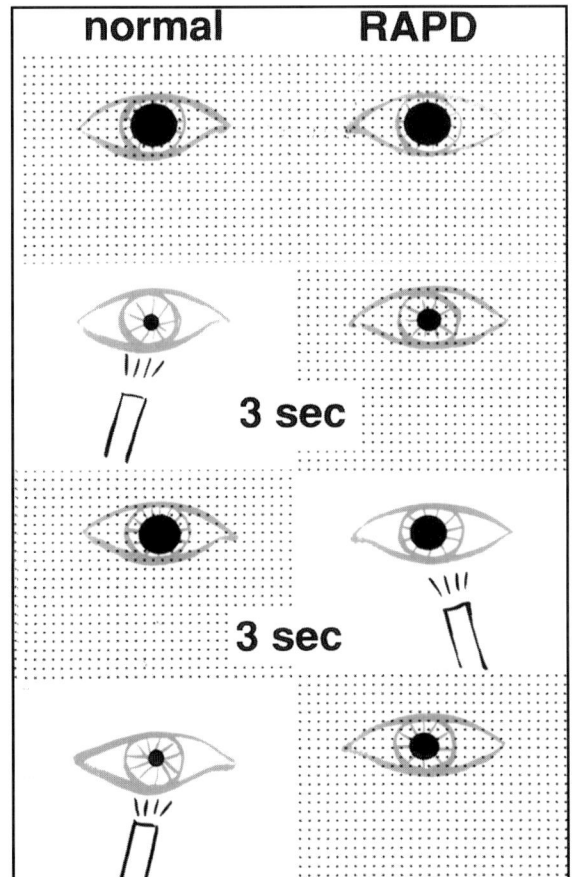

Figure 4.5. The swinging flash light test [55]. Top row: The patient is placed in dim light – both pupils show dilatation. Second row: Following direct light stimulation, the normal right eye exhibits a brisk pupillary constriction, and the unstimulated left eye shows a consensual response. Third row: The left eye is now tested – no pupillary constriction but merely dilatation is observed upon stimulation with direct light. Bottom row: Swinging the light back to the normal eye again produces a brisk direct (right) and a consensual left response.

left eye is tested. Red saturation is tested by pressing a finger on top of the light source.

Pupillary Function
The pupillary reactions allow for the most sensitive assessment of optic nerve dysfunction, and unlike visual acuity testing, pupillary function can be evaluated in the unconscious patient.

Optic-nerve dysfunction leads to a decrease of the direct pupillary reaction because of reduced afferent input into the pupillomotor system, while the consensual reaction remains intact (relative or incomplete afferent pupillary defect, RAPD). The clinical diagnosis is made with the swinging flash light test [54] (Figure 4.5)[4].

The test is performed in a dim room using a flashlight. The light is passed back and forth from under the right to the left eye at a frequency of 3 to 5 seconds, the pupillary response being closely observed.

In a normal eye the first reaction of each pupil to direct light stimulation is a brisk pupillary constriction, whereas in an eye with afferent pupillary defect, absence of constriction or even dilatation is observed when the light is directed toward the injured eye.

Anisocoria (fixed unilateral dilated pupil) is usually not due to trauma to the optic nerve, but rather results from dysfunction of the efferent pathway (third cranial nerve). Testing for a RAPD is more difficult under these conditions.

Testing for Double Vision
Double vision is not a reason for immediate intervention. It is, however, an indicator for the severity of the trauma and makes CT evaluation necessary, should it not rapidly subside.

Because of the often life-threatening condition of the emergency patient, evaluation of the visual system is easily forgotten. ROA (rapid ophthalmologic assessment), however, may save vision in a number of patients.

Management of Traumatic Visual Loss

Globe Injury

Every injury to the globe must be examined and treated immediately by an ophthalmic surgeon.

Because of the sparse vascularization of the globe, immunological resistance is low, and lacerations carry a high risk of infection. Immediate repair is therefore mandatory and must be done before any fracture repair is undertaken. The prognosis for visual recovery after repair of open-globe injuries depends largely on the severity of the initial trauma. Impaired visual acuity and a relative afferent pupillary defect on admission indicate a poor prognosis [56].

Traumatic Optic Neuropathy

This term stands for a group of pathological conditions[5] with different treatment requirements. In the past, therapeutic recommendations were contradictory, ranging from observation [57] to unrestricted surgical therapy [58].

At present, there are widely accepted indications for immediate decompressive surgery as well as a consensus for therapy with mega-dose corticosteroids and possible subsequent surgery [59-61]. A strategy for therapeutic decision making is shown in the flowchart in Figure 4.6.

Immediate Surgery
Immediate decompressive surgery is indicated in the following situations (Nos. 1 and 2 in flowchart):
1) *Progressive visual loss or deterioration of visual function after a lucid interval:* Prior to surgery, a CT scan is performed to detect a possible retrobulbar hematoma, bony fractures, or optic nerve sheath enlargement. If none of these can be found, compression of the nerve in the optic canal by hematoma or edema is assumed, and decompression is directed to the canal [62] (see below for technique).
2) Complete visual loss at presentation, if the CT scan shows one of the following surgically treatable pathologies:
   - retrobulbar or subperiosteal hematoma;
   - blow-in fractures with obvious constriction of orbital volume;
   - optic nerve-sheath enlargement.

Retrobulbar hematoma and large blow-in fractures have already been mentioned as mechanisms causing visual loss. Pain and globe proptosis are clinical signs indicating elevated intraorbital pressure, with the CT scan confirming the diagnosis. Depending on the situation, drainage or open reduction is necessary to achieve decompression. There is a good prognosis for visual recovery in retrobulbar hematoma [43, 48, 63, 64] as well as in blow-in fractures [65, 66].

Optic nerve-sheath enlargement, detectable with CT examination or ultrasonography [53], is another surgically treatable condition [67, 68]. Optic nerve-sheath decompression is performed by an ophthalmic surgeon via a medial orbitotomy.

There is controversy about the indications for immediate surgery in patients with visual loss and fractures running through the optic canal, because the prognosis is usually poor. Nevertheless, recovery of some vision is possible, and surgery should be offered to these patients.

It must be mentioned, however, that a fracture running through the optic canal is not per se an indication for decompressive surgery – if it is not associated with visual loss. The patient should receive mega-dose corticosteroids to reduce edema and meticulous monitoring of visual acuity is necessary (see Case 4.5).

Mega-Dose Corticosteroids
In the absence of a pathologic CT finding indicating immediate surgery, patients with impaired visual acuity are treated with mega-dose corticosteroids (No. 3 in flowchart). Although not yet proven in a controlled double-blind study, several authors have shown a positive effect of steroids on visual recovery [59, 63, 67], paralleling findings in spine injury [60].

In order to be effective, the dosage must be above a certain threshold [61]. An accepted protocol is given below:

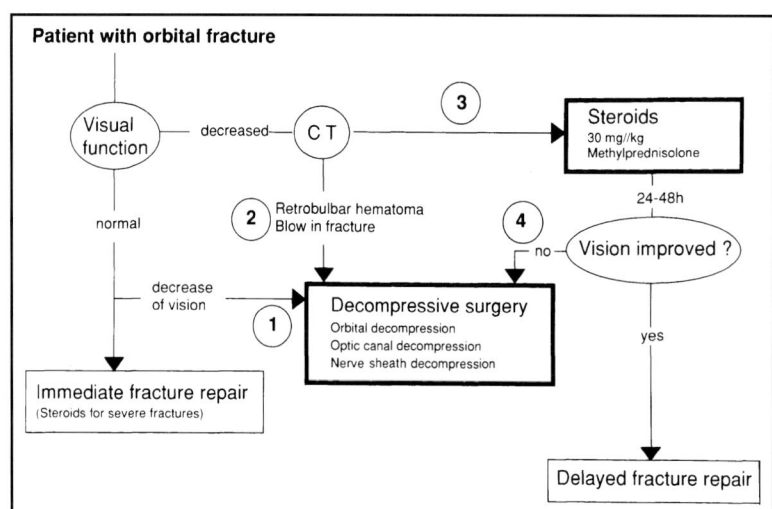

Figure 4.6. Decision making for decompressive surgery in patients with traumatic visual loss. See text for explanation.

Steroid treatment [53]
Loading dose:
– Methylprednisolone 30 mg/kg within 15 min.
– after 2 hours: 15 mg/kg
Maintenance dosage:
– Methylprednisolone 15 mg/kg every 6 hours

If there is no effect after 24 to 48 hours of corticosteroid administration, decompression of the optic canal should be offered to the patient (No. 4 in flowchart). A positive effect of optic-canal decompression has been shown as late as 5 days after the onset of blindness [69].

Technique of Optic Canal Decompression
Decompression of the intracanalicular optic nerve involves removal of the roof or medial wall of the optic canal; this can be performed via a transcranial or subcranial route. Subcranial optic-nerve decompression may be accomplished via transantral [70], endoscopic transnasal [71], or external ethmoidectomy approaches [72], the choice depending on a personal preference and one's experience with the respective techniques required. Familiar with craniofacial techniques, the first author uses a modified ethmoidectomy approach with superior orbital marginotomy (see also Section 7.1, Figure 7.7).

Visual Loss Following Fracture Repair

Visual loss following repair of orbital fractures is a rare but very severe complication [73, 74, 75]. The mechanism may be retrobulbar hemorrhage, increased intraorbital pressure due to excessive antral packing [74], or direct injury to the optic nerve from a displaced bone graft.

Visual function should be routinely tested after every orbital fracture repair. If there are any abnormal findings, emergency ophthalmologic consultation as well as CT scans must be obtained.

Any surgically treatable pathology requires immediate intervention.

Case Reports

Case 4.1

Complete visual loss from retrobulbar hematoma. This 48-year-old patient with a nondisplaced left zygomatico-orbital fracture had no light perception (NLP) on admission. Severe pain and proptosis was present in the left eye. The CT scan showed multiple hemorrhage into the retrobulbar cone (Figure 4.2).

Within 4 hours, decompression of the orbit was performed via a lower eyelid incision. A small hematoma could be evacuated, and a bleeding vessel arising from the infraorbital artery was coagulated.

The day after surgery, finger counting was possible; 3 months later, visual acuity was restored to 1.0.

Case 4.2

Visual loss associated with a blow-in fracture. A 45-year-old patient was struck in the right fronto-temporal area by a large wooden chest, causing a frontal skull fracture and bilateral orbital fractures, the left orbital fracture being a large blow-in fracture (Figure 4.3). He was fully conscious on admission, and rapid ophthalmologic assessment was normal on both eyes. Shortly after CT examination, the visual acuity in the left eye dramatically deteriorated, and 2 hours after the accident there was total loss of light perception in the left eye.

The patient was operated on within 6 hours of the accident, decompression of the left orbit being accomplished via a coronal approach with a superior marginotomy. A small hematoma was evacuated, and the displaced medial wall fragment was removed. No optic-canal decompression was performed. Bilateral orbital reconstruction was performed in the same operation.

Immediately after surgery, light perception was noted by the patient, and rapid improvement of visual acuity up to 1.0 occurred in the following 3 months.

Nevertheless, double vision was still present 11 months after trauma, most likely of neurogenic origin (cranial nerve IV).

Case 4.3

Visual loss without evident findings. After being hit by a car, a 49-year-old man was admitted to the hospital with a Glasgow coma score of 11, which improved to 15 within 3 days, at which time he complained about blindness in his left eye. The CT examination showed no surgically treatable pathology. The patient was immediately treated with cortico-

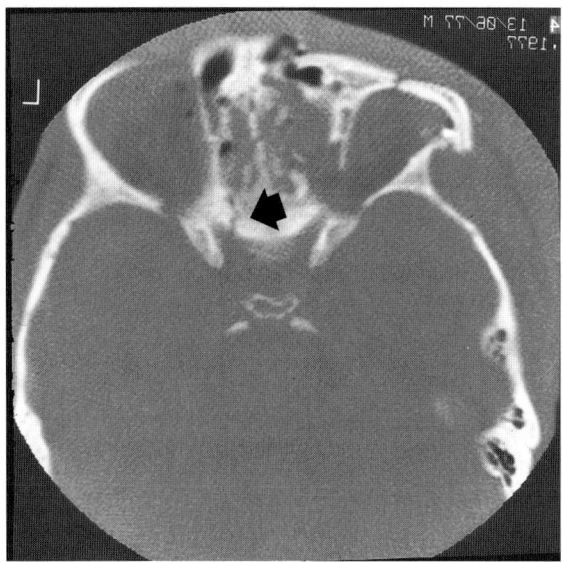

Figure 4.7. Fracture of the optic canal (Case 4.5). A fracture line running through the left optic canal (arrow), without visual impairment (same patient as shown in Figure 7.27).

steroids (standard dosage was methylprednisolone 500 mg/day at that time), and decompression of the optic canal via a modified ethmoidectomy approach was performed on the fourth day after the injury.

Despite therapy, complete visual loss remained unchanged.

Case 4.4

Visual loss associated with optic-canal fracture. A 23-year-old patient sustained a right orbital fracture with complete visual loss on admission. CT evaluation showed a fracture of the roof of the optic canal. Twenty-four hours after the accident, transcranial optic canal decompression was performed by a neurosurgeon.

After the operation, the patient still had no light perception in the right eye. Improvement to a visual acuity of 0.2 (finger count at 30 cm) took place within 8 weeks and then remained stable.

Case 4.5

Optic-canal fracture without visual loss (Figure 4.7). An 18-year-old patient sustained an open brain injury with complex right orbital fracture, skull-base fracture, and a fracture line running through the left optic canal.

The patient was unconscious on admission, but the swinging flash light test was normal. High-dose steroids were administered, and immediate repair of the dura as well as the right orbit and the skull was performed.

Despite severe contamination, uneventful healing took place, with vision 1.0 in both eyes and double vision present only in extreme gaze to the right. (same patient as in Case 7.5).

4.2 Diplopia

Double vision causes the patient to see the same object at two different places in space. In the early posttraumatic and postoperative period, it is a common complaint that usually resolves or improves considerably within days or weeks. A number of orbital fractures, however, are complicated by persisting diplopia, which, once established, may be difficult to correct.

Mechanisms

There are three principal mechanisms causing diplopia in trauma cases:

Edema and Hematoma

In the early posttraumatic or postoperative period, a change of the position of the globe as well as impairment of motility secondary to edema and hematoma often results in diplopia. This condition rapidly improves with the resolution of edema, though a slight motility disorder leading to double vision in extreme positions of gaze may persist for several months.

Restrictive Motility Disorder (Mechanical)

This condition is often associated with unrepaired or inadequately repaired orbital fractures. Trauma to the orbit leads not only to bone defects, but also causes disruption of the periorbit with soft tissue herniation into the maxillary and ethmoid sinus. Inadequate orbital reconstruction with residual herniation of soft tissues causes the delicate intraorbital

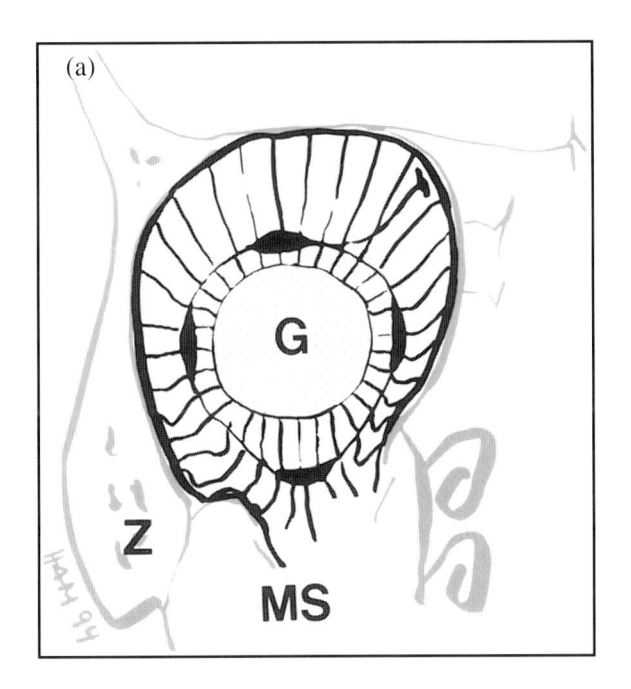

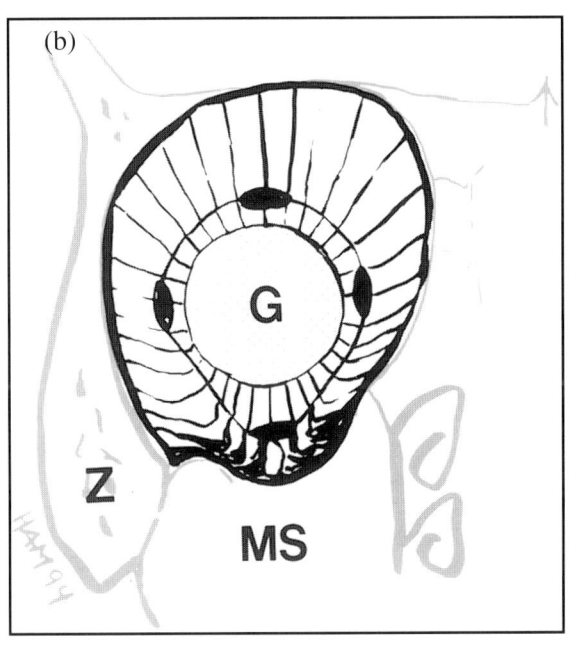

Figure 4.8 (a, b). Schematic cross-section of the right orbit. (a) Trauma to the orbit not only leads to defects in the orbital walls, but also causes disruption of the periorbit and the delicate intraorbital ligament system. (b) Inadequate repair causes the ligament system to heal in a distorted position which favors adhesions between individual ligaments as well as between the periorbit and the ligament system, resulting in restrictive motility disorder. G: ocular globe, Z: Zygomatic body, MS: maxillary sinus (redrawn after Koorneef [77], with permission).

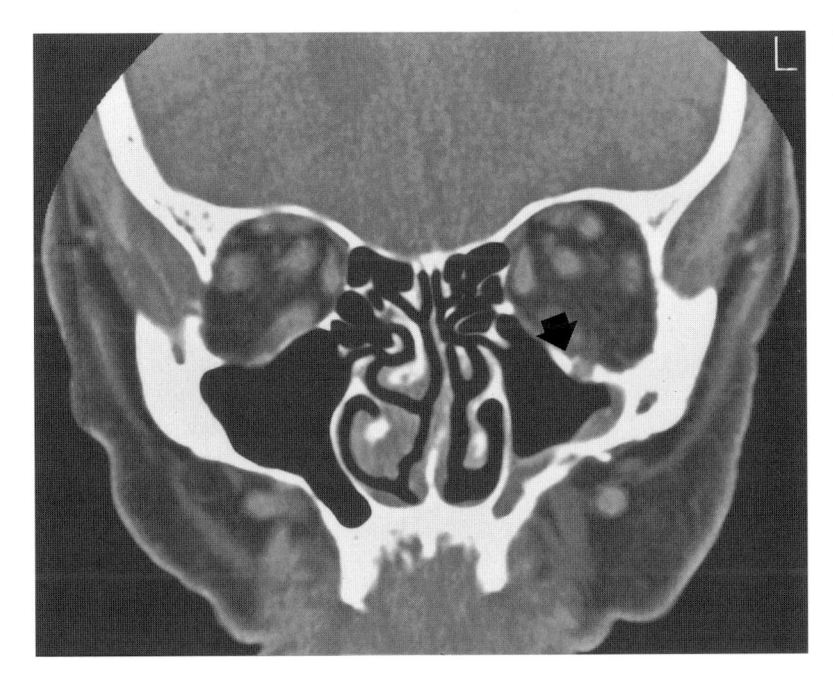

Figure 4.9. Coronal CT scan of a patient suffering from restricted downward gaze 6 months after a linear fracture of the left orbital floor. The soft tissue window demonstrates adhesions between inferior rectus muscle and periorbit (arrow).

ligament system [76] to heal in a distorted position with adhesions forming inside the ligament system itself, as well as between the ligament system and periorbit [77] (Figure 4.8).

Restrictive motility disorders are typically associated with orbital fractures of greater severity. Yet, minor defects and even linear fractures may cause adhesions [77] (Figure 4.9).

These findings underline the importance of early orbital fracture repair.

Diplopia caused by direct entrapment of extraocular muscles [32, 78] usually presents with vertical diplopia. However, muscle entrapment seems to be less frequent than previously postulated [77].

Cranial Nerve Injury (Neurogenic)

Functional impairment of the cranial nerves (most often the sixth cranial nerve) may result from direct (hematoma/dislocated fragments causing compression) or indirect (acceleration/deceleration) trauma, the latter even occurring in blunt head trauma without evidence of fractures. The differentiation from restrictive disorders is important because of the therapeutic possibilities offered by botulinum toxin injections (see below).

A large number of cranial nerve palsies spontaneously recover either completely or partially, within 6 to 9 months. The rate of recovery shows some correlation with the severity of the initial deficit.

The functional disturbances caused by diplopia range from negligible to severe. Binocular vision in straight and downward gaze (for reading) is most important for activities of daily living. Double vision in upward gaze, as well as in the left and right direction, is of minor importance in daily life, though it may interfere with driving. Diplopia in extreme fields of gaze is a negligible disorder.

The complex nature of diplopia is evident from the fact that many patients are able to maintain binocular single vision except when tired. This observation demonstrates the importance of the central nervous system component.

Diagnosis and Documentation

The diagnostic evaluation of patients complaining of posttraumatic diplopia includes orbital CTs as well as ophthalmologic consultation and follow-up.

CTs of the orbit in axial and coronal planes allow detection of residual defects in the orbital walls. Adhesions and herniations may be detected with the soft tissue window.

Cooperation with an ophthalmologist is of utmost importance. In the initial phase, exact and reproducible documentation as well as accurate diagnosis permits assessment of the severity of the motility disorder as well as the documentation of spontaneous improvement. Symptomatic therapy helps the patient to master daily life.

Moreover, an in-depth diagnosis is necessary to distinguish between the different etiologies of diplopia, and to decide about the timing and types of active therapy. Basic diagnostic tests are described below:

The Corneal Light Reflex
This test permits assessment of the relative position of the eyes.

Testing Ductions, Versions and Saccadic Velocity
The eye movements, with the patient following the finger in all 8 directions of gaze, are examined to detect limitations of excursions. Testing for saccadic velocity can provide subtle information in cases of partial cranial nerve palsy, especially when compared to the contralateral eye (dissociated nystagmus).

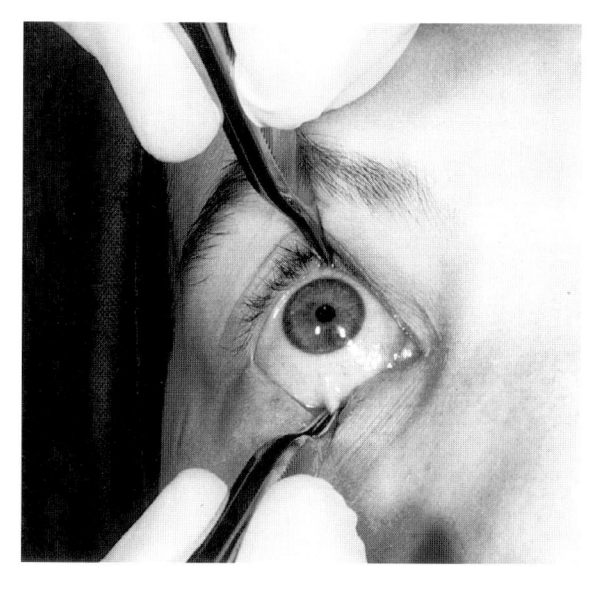

Figure 4.10. Forced duction test. The forced duction test permits assessment of the passive motility of the globe. It is performed with the help of two fine forceps. One forceps is used to seize the conjunctiva near the muscle insertion, while the other one stabilizes the eye during the pickup procedure.

Forced Duction Test (Figure 4.10)
The forced duction test evaluates the passive motility of the globe. In the normal eye, there is virtually no resistance against passive motion.

This test is helpful for distinguishing between restrictive and neurogenic motility disorders. Moreover, it is a basic maneuver necessary to exclude impingement of soft tissues between grafts and or-

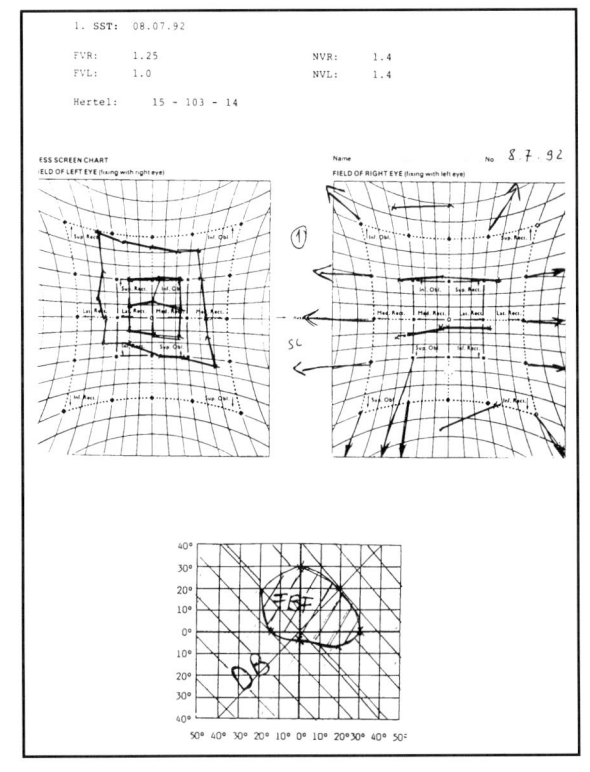

Figure 4.11. Documentation of eye motility disorders and visual field with the Hess chart and the field of binocular vision. The Hess chart (top) shows limited motility of the left eye in all directions of gaze. The field of binocular vision is restricted (bottom).

bital walls during reconstruction of the internal orbit (see Section 7.5).

Electromyography
Electromyograpy of the extraocular muscles is the method of choice for further evaluation of neurogenic disorders. An electrode needle is stuck into the muscle in question under local anesthesisa and the signals are recorded. In order to test recruitment, the patient is asked to look into the direction of action of the paretic eye muscle, this maneuver allowing for the greatest level of recruitment. If only a reduced signal – or no signal at all – can be recorded, the paretic nature of the condition is evident.

Hess Screen/Binocular Field of Vision
Documentation and follow-up of double vision is most efficiently done with the Hess screen and the binocular field of vision (Figure 4.11).

The Hess screen gives information about the extent and type of motility disorder by measuring the incomitance pattern [79]. Its quantitative nature and reproducibility make it a powerful follow-up tool. Limitations of motility are well demonstrated, which facilitates communication between ophthalmologist and nonophthalmologist.

In addition, it allows the experienced ophthalmologist to differentiate between different etiologies of motility problems.

The binocular field of vision directly demonstrates the areas of gaze where the patient has binocular vision.

Management

Motility disorders of neurogenic origin as well as disorders caused by edema may spontaneously improve within the first 6–8 months. Therefore, in the inital period after trauma, management is essentially symptomatic in order to help the patient with activities of daily living. Recording diplopia with the Hess screen and field of binocular vision permits correct follow-up.

The therapeutic spectrum includes conservative measures, botulinum toxin injections, and strabismus surgery. An algorithm for management of patients with diplopia is shown in Figure 4.12.

Figure 4.12. Management of posttraumatic diplopia (see text for explanations).

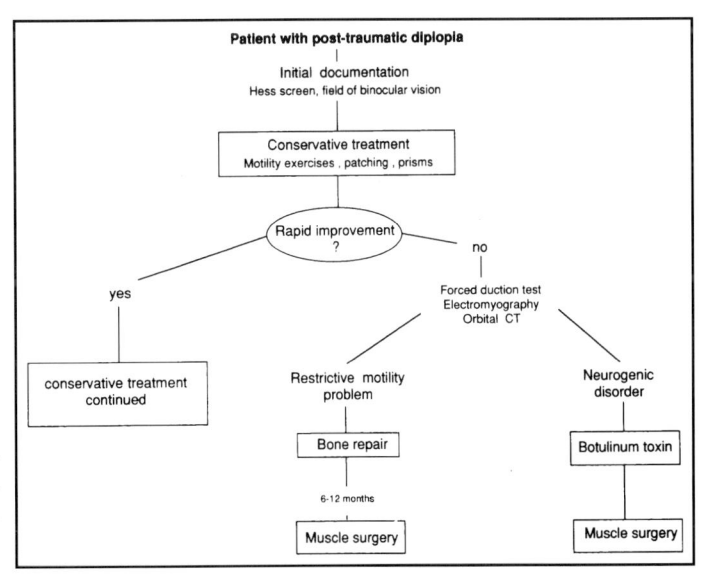

Conservative Treatment

Conservative treatment should begin immediately after trauma or bone surgery and is essentially symptomatic. The main elements are:

Motility Exercises
They should be started immediately in every patient complaining of double vision, even if no deviation of the eyes can be detected by gross examination. The patient is asked to move the eyes in all directions of gaze, especially the direction in which the double image tends to separate most. This simple measure helps to prevent adhesions of soft tissue structures within the orbit.

OcclusionTherapy
Occlusion of one eye immediately frees the patient from double vision, but also reduces the visual field dramatically. This therapy can be recommended as an initial measure in all patients complaining of disturbing diplopia without regard to the underlying pathophysiology of double vision.

Press-on Prisms
When the angle of deviation is not exeedingly large, eyeglasses with press-on prisms may restore a field of binocular vision in straight gaze. The degree of correction can easily be adapted to the gradual spontaneous improvement of eye motility. Prisms may eventually be utilized to definitely correct a mild residual diplopia in straight gaze.

Botulinum Toxin Injections

Many neuro-ophthalmic units recommend early botulinum toxin treatment for diplopia of neurogenic origin [80–82]. The toxin is injected into the ipsilateral direct antagonist of the paretic muscle. It has been shown to accelerate the restoration of binocular vision by dampening the so-called "muscle sequelae"[6].

Botulinum toxin injections were helpful in two of our patients with neurogenic motility disorders [84].

Surgical Therapy

The function of the extraocular muscles can surgically be influenced in the following ways:

Weakening Procedures
The action of an extraocular muscle is weakened by recessing the muscle behind its original insertion. This procedure is usually used in the case of excessive function of the ipsilateral antagonist of an impaired muscle. In restrictive motility disorders, weakening of the contralateral synergist reduces double vision by limiting excursions in a given direction.

Strengthening Procedures
Shortening of a muscle by partial resection increases the tension at rest and the resultant force of contraction. The procedure is useful to improve the action of partially paretic muscles. Prior to surgery, a total paresis of the muscle to be corrected should be excluded with electromyography.

Muscle Transpositions
This procedure consists of a transposition of half a muscle belly from agonist muscles to the insertion of a paretic muscle. An example is the transposition of the inferior and superior rectus muscles to replace a paretic lateral rectus muscle.

Eye muscle surgery should be delayed for at least 6 months after the accident or the last reconstructive procedure to allow for a maximum of spontaneous recovery.

An anatomically reconstructed orbit is the basis for eye muscle surgery, and therefore all reconstructive osseous procedures must be performed first (first the bone, then the soft tissues).

Chapter 5
Conservative Treatment

There has been a long-standing controversy about conservative versus operative management of orbital fractures. Since Converse's classic papers advocating early repair of orbital fractures [32, 85, 86], surgeons preferring operative treatment have debated with authors favoring a conservative approach, the most often cited one among them being Putterman [87].

Before the introduction of CT scanning, an exact description of fracture patterns was not possible; therefore, different fractures were compared to each other. Today, reliable criteria for conservative or operative management of orbital fractures have been formulated [88].

Conservative treatment may be considered in a small subset of orbital fractures (3% in our own patients, see Table 6.1.9): those without dislocation of the orbital frame, and blow-out fractures limited to a single orbital wall without diplopia or with rapidly resolving diplopia (Figure 5.1).

Possible sequelae of neglected orbital fractures include persistent diplopia and enophthalmos, both of these being conditions that may be difficult to correct secondarily. The decision for conservative management should therefore be made with deliberation. It is important to note that enophthalmos often develops as a late symptom, initially masked by swelling.

Specific contraindications against conservative treatment include the following conditions:
- Dislocated fractures of the orbital frame.
- Clinically detectable enophthalmos or vertical globe distopia.
- Severe restriction of the eye motility (forced duction test), indicating incarceration of soft tissues.

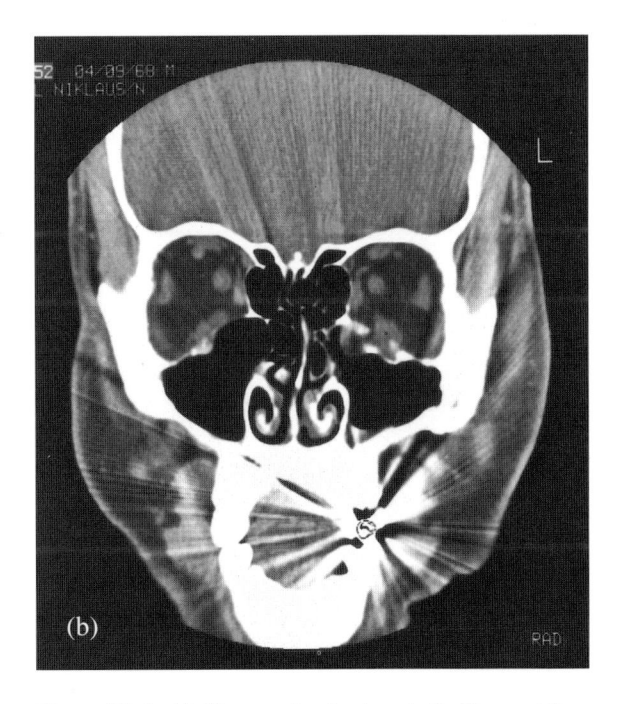

Figure 5.1 (a, b). Conservative treatment of a blow-out fracture. Axial (a) and coronal (b) scans of a blow-out fracture limited to the left orbital floor. Inital double vision improved rapidly; after 6 months, normal binocular vision was documented and no enophthalmos was present.

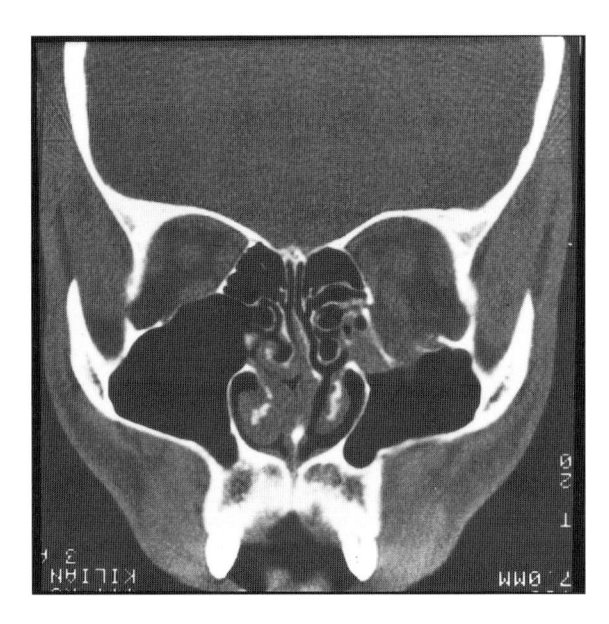

Figure 5.2. Conservative treatment not indicated. A fracture of the left orbital floor with considerable soft-tissue herniation into the maxillary sinus. The patient initially suffered from double vision, which rapidly improved, and he refused operative repair. A 3 mm enophthalmos was present after 7 months. (This patient was treated in 1987 and he is therefore not included in the review presented in Chapter 6.)

- Fractures involving several orbital walls, thus creating considerable volume enlargement.
- Fractures of the orbital floor extending posteriorly into the key area (Figure 5.2) or causing enlargement of the infraorbital fissure.

In order to minimize the damage to any incarcerated soft tissues, operative treatment should be undertaken as early as possible. Manson [88] claims that, with the combined insult of trauma and surgery, the closer the events are in time, the less the injury to the soft tissues, thus favoring immediate surgery. According to our own clinical impression, immediate surgery produces less swelling than delayed treatment, the reason for which is not entirely clear to us.

Elevated intracranial pressure may be a contraindication against immediate surgery in severely injured patients. Yet with the modern possibility of CT and continuous intracranial pressure monitoring, a head injury per se does not represent a contraindication against immediate surgery [89].

Chapter 6
Database

The data presented in this chapter represent a review of patients with orbital fractures treated at the University Hospital Basel, Switzerland, and the County Hospital of Aarau, Switzerland. The patients in both hospitals were operated on by staff of the Clinic for Reconstructive Surgery of the University Hospital Basel, the majority of the complex fractures (65%) being operated on by the author.

Additionally, a review of patients who underwent secondary corrections by the author is included.

6.1 Review of Patients with Primary Repair

Patient Population

Between January 1988 and December 1992, 513 patients with fractures involving the orbits were treated primarily in the above-mentioned hospitals (Table 6.1.1). Sixty-five patients were excluded from the review because of inadequate records and/or loss of follow-up. The remaining 448 patients (87%) were followed for a minimum of 6 months (see below for follow-up protocol). The high follow-up rate was attained because most of the patients live within a 100-km radius of the hospitals, and because the Swiss insurance system (which includes foreign workers in the country) requires continued after-care [27].

The age distribution (Figure 6.1) exhibits a peak between 20 and 30 years, resulting from the increased readiness of members of this age group to take risks, especially when driving motor vehicles. There was a male to female preponderance of 3.3:1. The percentage of complex fracture patterns decreases in the older patients, since these patients are no longer involved in work-related accidents. Traffic accidents, mostly car accidents, were the prevalent

Table 6.1.1. Patients with orbital fractures 1988–1992.

Patients treated	513	100%
Excluded (inadequate records/ lack of follow-up)	65	13%
Patients reviewed	448	87%

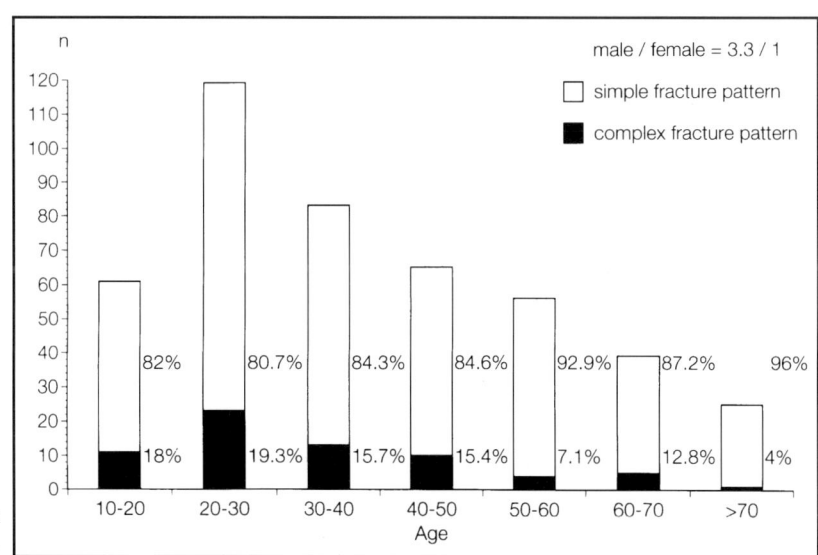

Figure 6.1. Age and sex distribution of 448 patients with orbital fractures.

Table 6.1.2. Causes of orbital fractures in 448 patients.

Cause	No. patients	%
Traffic accident	175	39%
Work-related accident	40	9%
Sports	63	14%
Violence	54	12%
Housework	40	9%
Miscellaneous	76	17%
Total	448	100%

Table 6.1.3. Number of orbital fractures in 448 patients.

	No. patients	No. fractures
Unilateral fractures	364	364
Bilateral fractures	84	168
Total	448	532

cause (Table 6.1.2), accounting for 39% of the fractures.

Fracture Patterns and Associated Injuries

Distribution of Fracture Patterns

The 448 patients had a total of 532 orbital fractures, 84 (18%) of the patients sustaining bilateral orbital fractures (Table 6.1.3).

The distribution of fracture sites is shown in Figure 6.2. Orbito-zygomatic fractures constitute the largest group (76%). Defects of the orbital walls were mostly associated with orbital frame injuries. Only 2.8% of the fractures presented as isolated orbital-wall injuries.

The majority of orbito-zygomatic injuries consisted of single-piece fractures (Type I, see Chapter 3 for classification), occasionally with an infraorbital fragment and or an anterior orbital floor defect (Type III) (Table 6.1.4), closed reduction or stabilization via local incisions being the usual management. In our series, only 17 (4%) of the isolated orbito-zygomatic fractures were classified as truly complex, whereas other authors have found 12% [90], 18% [26], and even 35% [27] of fractures to be comminuted. It is difficult to determine whether these figures express a real difference in the fracture patterns or merely in the definition of fragmentation.

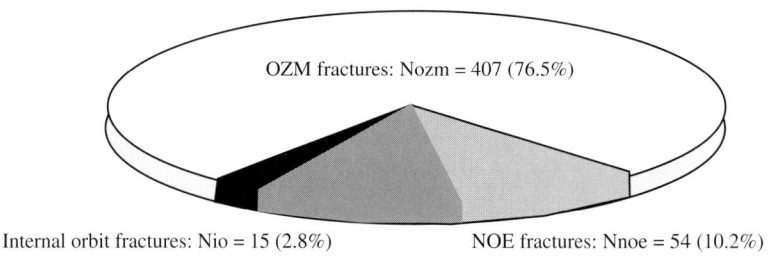

Figure 6.2. Distribution of fracture sites in 532 orbital fractures. OZM: Orbito-zygomatic fractures, NOE: Naso-orbito-ethmoid fractures.

OZM fractures: Nozm = 407 (76.5%)
Internal orbit fractures: Nio = 15 (2.8%)
NOE fractures: Nnoe = 54 (10.2%)
Combined fractures: Ncf = 56 (10.5%)

Table 6.1.4. Distribution of fracture patterns in 407 orbito-zygomatic (OZM) fractures, constituting 76% of all 532 orbital fractures (classification see Chapter 3).

Type of OZM fracture	Description	No. fract.	% of 407
Type I	undisplaced or minimally displaced	179	44%
Type II	segmental	17	4%
Type III	displaced, infraorbital fragment, frequently floor fracture	194	48%
Type IV	comminuted, associated with complex wall defects	17	4%
Total		407	100%

Table 6.1.5. Distribution of fracture patterns in 54 naso-orbito-ethmoid (NOE) fractures, constituting 10% of all 532 orbital fractures (classification see Chapter 3).

Type of NOE fracture	Description	No. fract.	% of 54
Type I	nonfragmented, large central fragment	40	75%
Type II	fragmentation, sizeable central fragment	2	3%
Type III	severe fragmentation, no sizeable central fragment	12	22%
Total		54	100%

The majority of naso-orbito-ethmoid fractures exhibited a single canthal-ligament-bearing fragment (Table 6.1.5), though an extended approach was frequently utilized to ensure correct reduction of the fragment.

Associated Injuries

Facial and head injuries associated with orbital fractures are listed in Table 6.1.6, the most important among them being cerebral[7] and ocular injuries. Table 6.1.7 shows the mechanisms for traumatic visual loss.

Table 6.1.6. Associated facial and head injuries in 448 patients with orbital fractures.

Type of injury	No. patients	% of 448
Maxillary fractures	49	11%
Mandibular fractures	25	6%
Cerebral injury*	27	6%
Skull base	16	4%
Frontal sinus	20	5%
Nasal injury	46	10%
Visual loss**	23	5%
Total patients with associated facial and head injuries	206	47%

* Closed head injury (CHI) without morphologic findings is not included.
** See Table 6.1.7 for mechanisms.

Table 6.1.7. Mechanisms of complete visual loss in 23 (5%) of 448 patients with orbital fractures.

Mechanism	No. patients	% of 23
Globe rupture/avulsion	12	52%
Retrobulbar hematoma	3	13%
Optic canal fracture	3	13%
Unknown etiology	5	22%
Total patients with visual loss	23	100%

Complete visual loss on admission or immediately thereafter was present in 23 patients (5%), with globe rupture being the most frequent cause (Table 6.1.7). All patients except for one had no light perception on admission, the exception being a patient with a severe blow-in fracture and retrobulbar hematoma presenting with full vision which then decreased to no light perception within 2 hours (Case 4.2, Chapter 4).

Associated injuries not involving the head or face are listed in Table 6.1.8, the most frequent among them being orthopedic fractures. There was only a single isolated abdominal injury associated with or-

Table 6.1.8. Associated injuries (except facial and head) in 448 patients with orbital fractures.

Type of injury	No. patients	% of 448
Chest	7	2%
Abdominal	1	0%
Orthopedic	31	7%
Spine	3	1%
Polytrauma	14	3%
Total associated injuries	56	13%

bital fractures, whereas 8 of the 14 polytrauma patients had abdominal injuries.

Operative Treatment

Early primary repair was undertaken as soon as possible: 76% of the patients were operated on within the first 72 hours after the accident. A number of minor fractures (21%) were delayed for logistical reasons, whereas in 3% of patients, neurologic and/or anesthesiologic problems contraindicated early surgery.

Type of Repair

Table 6.1.9 summarizes the type of treatment given during the entire period of observation. With regard to operative management, there has been a significant increase in the application of craniofacial techniques from 1988 to 1992 (Figure 6.3). Miniplate fixation using the AO craniofacial system was the standard technique for the stabilization of orbital frame fractures.

Table 6.1.9. Treatment of 448 patients with orbital fractures during the years 1988 to 1992. (In patients with bilateral fractures treated with different approaches, the more extended approach took precedence in their classification.)

Treatment	No. patients	% of 448
Conservative	15	3%
Closed reduction	74	17%
Local incisions	265	59%
Extended approach	94	21%
Total	448	100%

In 237 (44.5%) of the 532 orbital fractures, some type of grafting was performed to reconstruct the internal orbit (Table 6.1.10): 74 bone grafts were used to bridge orbital-wall defects, mostly in complex fractures, and 137 fractures were reconstructed with alloplastic materials. The high number of

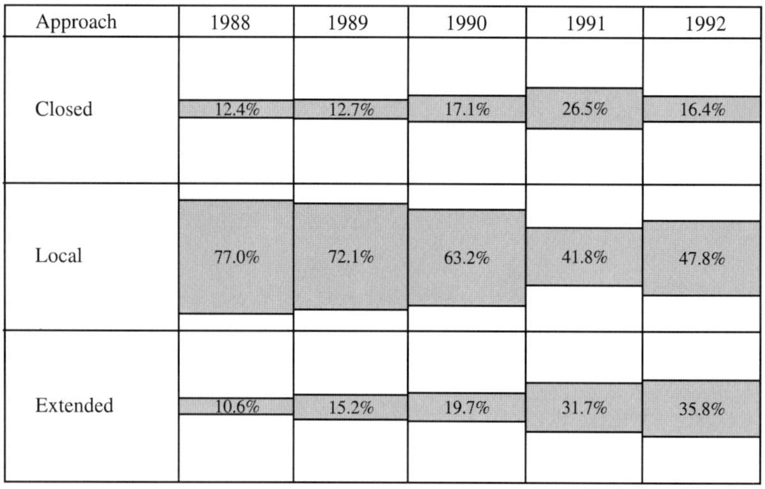

Approach	1988	1989	1990	1991	1992
Closed	12.4%	12.7%	17.1%	26.5%	16.4%
Local	77.0%	72.1%	63.2%	41.8%	47.8%
Extended	10.6%	15.2%	19.7%	31.7%	35.8%

Figure 6.3. Evolution of the operative approach from 1988 to 1992. During the years 1991 and 1992, there are more extended approaches than complex orbital fractures. This is because, in some cases, associated facial injuries required an extended approach (see Chapter 7). There has been a significant increase in extended approaches using craniofacial techniques.

Table 6.1.10. Materials and fixation techniques for the internal orbit used in 237 (45%) of 532 orbital fractures.

Fixation	Graft material	No. fractures	% of 532
No fixation	Osseous grafts		
	Rib	6	1%
	Calvaria	60	11%
	Iliac crest	8	1%
	Total bone grafts	74	13%
	Nonosseous grafts		
	Resorbable	43	8%
	Lyodura	77	15%
	Silastic	17	3%
	Total nonosseous	137	26%
Rigid fixation	Orbital plate	9	2%
	Cantilever graft	17	4%
	Total rigid fixation	26	6%
Total fractures grafted		237	45%

Rigid fixation techniques for the internal orbit [16] were used in our unit sporadically from 1988 to 1990 and have been in routine use since 1991. Their efficiency is underlined by the fact that only 2 (7%) of the 26 fractures reconstructed with rigid fixation developed enophthalmos, the overall incidence in the relevant fracture group being 18% (Table 6.1.14). And in these two patients, technical errors in the use of rigid fixation could be demonstrated (see Figure 7.5).

Adjunctive procedures were nasal reconstruction using calvarial bone grafts (18 cases) and medial canthopexy (25 cases).

The management and outcome of the patients presenting with visual loss is discussed in Section 6.1.5.

grafts results from our philosophy that linear fractures or minimal defects remaining after reduction of orbito-zygomatic fractures should be lined with a small graft in order to avoid adhesions between the fracture gap and orbital connective tissue (see Chapter 4, Figure 4.9).

The most frequently utilized bone graft was calvaria, the advantages being its availability in the same operative field and the low morbidity associated with its harvest. From 1988 to 1991, lyophilized dura was the standard nonosseous graft. We have since discontinued its use because of the poor structural qualities. Presently, our preferred alloplastic implant material is resorbable polydioxanone (PDS Ethicon) [91], which is available in 0.25-mm and 0.5-mm thick sheets (Figure 7.20).

Follow-Up

All 448 patients included in the review had a minimal follow-up period of 6 months (mean 10.4 months, range 6 to 18 months). Two follow-up protocols were used:

– A routine protocol, consisting of a clinical and standard x-ray examination. Clinical examination included subjective complaints (pain, V2-nerve paresthesia, cold sensation) as well as cosmetic inspection for visible scars and contour deformities, particularly malar flattening. Binocular vision was assessed by having the patient follow a finger with the eyes, and enophthalmos measurment was done using the Hertel exophthalmometer. Plain x-ray examination with waters view pro-

Table 6.1.11. Complications and late sequelae in 247 (55%) of 448 patients with orbital fractures.

	No. compl./ sequelae	No. patients	% of 448
Early complications (< 4 weeks)	17	14	3.1%
Late complications (> 4 weeks)	59	53	11.8%
Minor sequelae	256	162	30%
Major sequelae	36	18	4%
Total	368	247	49%

Table 6.1.12. Early complications (up to 4 weeks postoperatively) in 14 (2.8 %) of 448 patients.

Type of complication	No. complications	No. patients	% of 448
General			
Deep vein thrombosis	3	3	0.6%
Local			
Hematoma	3	1	0.2%
Wound dehiscence	4	4	0.8%
Oro-antral fistula	2	2	0.4%
Eye motility disorder caused by bone fragment	2	1	0.2%
Eye motility disorder caused by bone graft	1	1	0.2%
Corneal infection (Herpes)	2	2	0.4%
Total	17	14	2.8%

jection confirmed repneumatization of the paranasal sinuses.
– An extended protocol for patients with major orbital injuries and for patients revealing complications during routine examination. The extended follow-up protocol included a clinical examination, high-resolution CT scanning of the orbits (usually coronal and axial), ophthalmologic follow-up including Hess screen and field of binocular vision, and photographic documentation. 106 patients were included into the extended follow-up protocol.

Table 6.1.11 shows the total number of complications and late sequelae encountered in the 448 patients (detailed in Tables 6.1.12 to 6.1.14). The total number of patients presenting with complications and sequelae 247 (= 55%) may seem high at first; however, it must be noted that minor sequelae without clinical significance are also included in the table, adding 30% to the total percentage of 55%.

Early Postoperative Complications

A total of 17 early complications in 14 (2.8%) of patients was documented (Table 6.1.12).

Deep vein thrombosis necessitating full-dose heparinization complicated the early postoperative course of 3 patients, two of whom subsequently developed a hematoma in the operative field – in one case severe enough to require evacuation. While low-dose heparin is routinely given in elective surgery, this is not the case in severely traumatized patients, who often suffer from coagulopathies due to excessive blood loss. The low rate of thrombosis (0.6%) seems to justify this policy. Patients with low-velocity injuries, however, should routinely receive low-dose heparin or another antithrombotic agent.

Two cases of oro-antral fistula were due to insufficient closure of an upper buccal sulcus incision overlying a defect in the anterior maxillary wall. We now prefer to bridge every bony defect greater than 5 mm in diameter in the anterior maxillary sinus wall.

Impairment of eye motility secondary to a unreduced lateral wall fragment occurred in 1 patient (Figure 6.4). After a first revision using local incisions, the problem remained unchanged, and another intervention became necessary. A malpositioned bone graft protruding into the orbit caused a severe motility disorder in another patient (Figure 7.6, Chapter 7). Postoperative CT examination, however, was not done until 6 weeks after surgery, so that early revision surgery was not performed. The patient revealed diplopia in straight gaze, though subjective complaints were minimal because the impaired eye was suppressed, and late revision surgery was refused by the patient.

Loss of vision complicating primary repair of orbital fractures [73-75, 92] did not occur in this group of patients[8], nor did infection – which has been reported as a possible early complication of orbital fractures [93, 94] – occur from 1988 to 1992. In 1993, however, a severe orbital infection resulting in monocular blindness complicated a conservatively treated blow-out fracture of the orbital floor.

Figure 6.4. Orbito-zygomatic fracture type IV with an isolated lateral wall fragment. Reduction was attempted with local incisions witout adequate reduction of the lateral wall. The isolated fragment produced restriction of lateral eye movement.

Late Complications and Sequelae

The late complications (> 4 weeks after surgery) are listed in Table 6.1.14. There were 59 late complications in 53 (11.8%) patients, the most frequent being infection. The traumatized frontal sinus is highly susceptible to infection, frequently occurring after a cold.

Ectropion of the lower lid is a disfiguring complication that is difficult to correct (Figure 6.5). It occurred in 3 patients and was associated with infection ensuing from screw loosening at the infraorbital plate. Lid shortening after a high subciliary approach was noted in 9 patients. The contraindications for this type of incision are discussed in Chapter 7.

Permanent frontal nerve palsy was noted in 3 patients, all of whom were operated on during the first 2 years of the observation period. No further frontal nerve injuries have occurred since we routinely approach the zygomatic arch within the temporal fat pad [95] (Figure 7.4). However, slight to moderate temporal hollowing is observed more often, in spite of efforts to avoid direct exposure of the temporal muscle.

Five patients complained of chronic headache that did not respond to any kind of local (injections) or general (analgesics) treatment. These patients had all suffered from severe concomitant cerebral injuries, so that the headache probably relates to the cerebral injury.

Lacrimal duct obstruction leading to epiphora was observed in 4 patients, whereas 2 patients suffered from dry eyes, requiring constant use of artificial tears.

With regard to late sequelae, esthetic deformities and functional problems were evaluated (Table 6.1.14). The follow-up revealed minor deformities in 162 (30%) patients, whereas 18 (4%) patients had

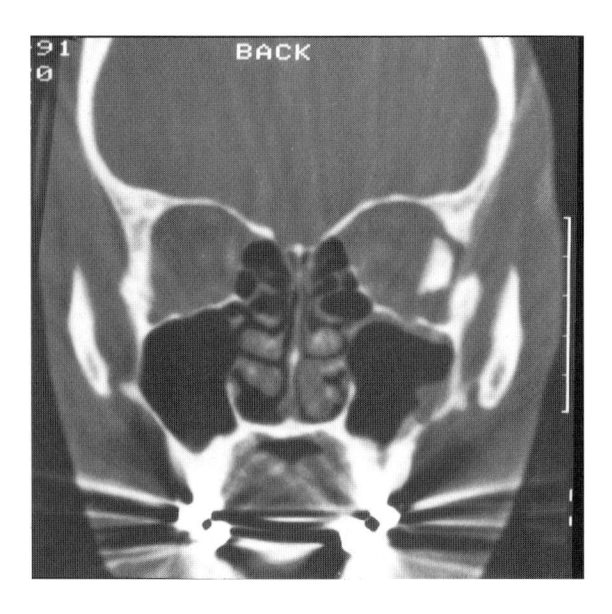

Table 6.1.13. Late complications (>4 weeks postoperative) in 53 (11.8%) of 448 patients.

Type of complication	No. complications	No. patients	% of 448
Infection originating from			
Screw loosening	11	11	
Silastic sheet	1	1	
Maxillary sinus	1	1	
Frontal sinus	12	6	
Total infections	25	19	4.2%
Plate exposure	8	8	1.7%
Permanant ectropion	3	3	0.6%
Lid shortening	9	9	2.0%
Epiphora	4	4	1.0%
Dry eye	2	2	0.5%
Frontal nerve palsy	3	3	0.6%
Chronic headache	5	5	1.1%
Total	59	53	11.8%

Table 6.1.14. Late deformities in 180 (34%) of 448 patients with orbital fractures.

	No. deform.	% of 532	No. patients	% of 448
Minor deformities				
Unfavourable scar	72			
Visible/palpable plate	103			
Minor malar asymmetry	58			
Mild enophthalmos (2 mm)	23			
Total minor deformities	256	48%	162	30%
Major (skeletal) deformities				
Eenophthalmos (>3 mm)	13			
Telecanthus (>38 mm)	11			
Malposition of zygoma	12			
Total major deformities	36	6%	18	4%
Total late deformities	292	54%	180	34%

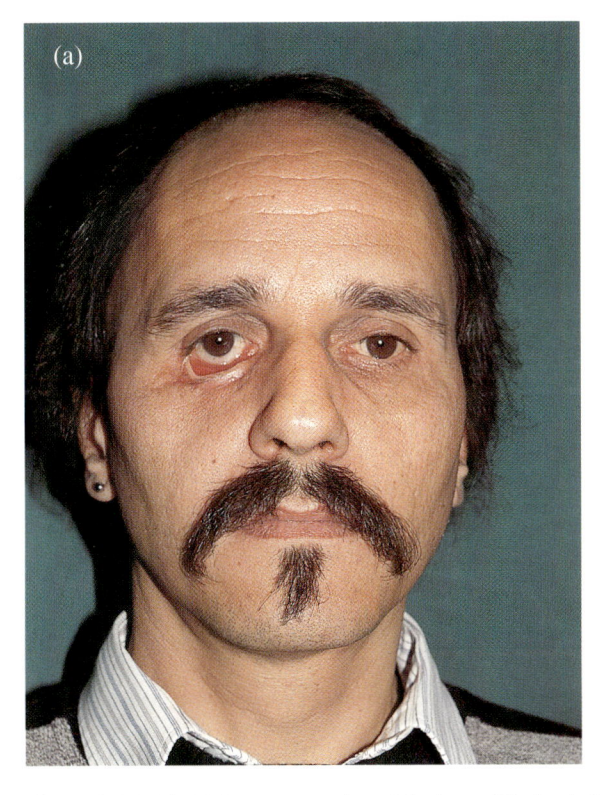

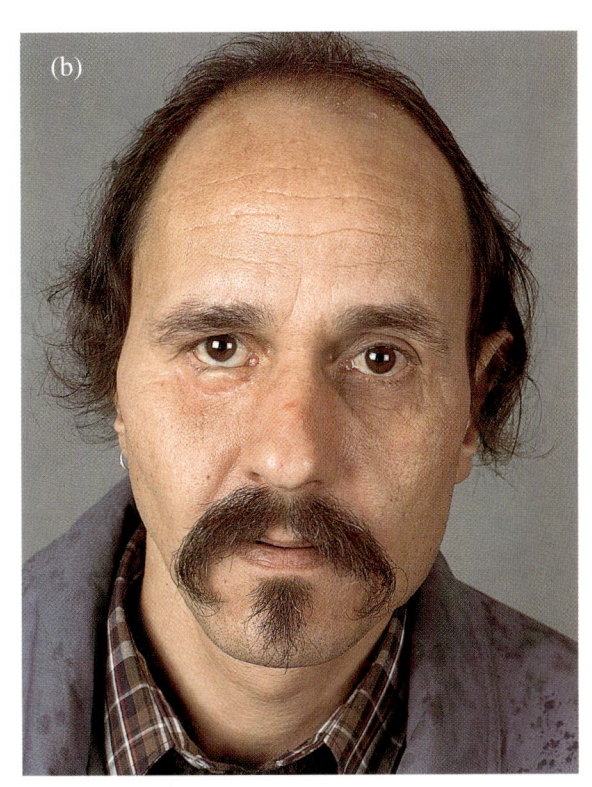

Figure 6.5 (a, b). (a) Severe ectropion of the lower lid after infection from screw loosening. (b) After two-stage correction using auricular cartilage graft and soft tissue suspension.

major skeletal deformities (examples: patients 8.1, 8.2 and 8.4 in Chapter 8).

Unfavorable scars were predominantly observed in the region of the lateral eyebrow. Instead of a lateral eyebrow incision, an upper blepharoplasty incision (Figure 7.1) is recommended.

Major deformities occurred exclusively as a sequel of complex fractures, enophthalmos being an important example:

Enophthalmos was defined as mild if the antero-posterior globe position between affected and unaffected eye differed by no more than 2 mm. Mild enophthalmos is not disfiguring (Figure 6.6), in fact the patients often hardly notice it. None of our patients with mild enophthalmos asked for corrective surgery. Differences of more than 3 mm or globe projection of less than 11 mm as measured with the Hertel exophthalmometer were defined as severe enophthalmos. Table 6.1.15 shows the frequency of enophthalmos as related to the fracture pattern.

Severe enophthalmos was observed only in complex fractures involving the deep orbit (Type IV orbito-zygomatic fractures and combined orbital fractures). In all cases of severe enophthalmos, residual defects in the posterior orbit could be found on CT examination, usually located in the posterior medial wall, defined as the key area (see Chapter 2). Technical errors in complex fracture repair are discussed in Section 7.5.

The importance of volumetric overcorrection in reconstructing the internal orbit cannot be overemphasized.

Functional Sequelae: Visual Loss and Diplopia

Table 6.1.16 shows the management and outcome of patients presenting with complete visual loss on admission. The prognosis was poor, except for patients with retrobulbar hematoma, all of whom recovered to normal visual acuity. The data do not allow any comment on the effect of optic canal decompression. The importance of early diagnosis must be pointed out in order to detect patients with a potentially excellent prognosis (retrobulbar hematoma), and to possibly improve the outcome of the other groups.

The diagnosis and management of visual impairment is discussed in Section 4.1.

Table 6.1.15. Enophthalmos at follow-up (minimum 6 months postoperatively) related to fracture pattern in 36 (7%) of 520 orbital fractures (532 minus 12 fractures, excluded for loss of eye or ptysis of globe). Significant enophthalmos (marked in gray) occurred exclusively as a sequel of complex fractures.

Fracture site	No. of patients excluded		Normal eye position		Mild enophth.		Severe enophth.		Total enophth.	
Internal orbit	15		14	(93%)	1	(6%)			1	(6%)
Orbito-zygomatic										
Type I	179		179	(100%)						
Type II	17		17	(17%)						
Type III	189	(5)	181	(96%)	8	(4.2%)			8	4.2%
Type IV	17		12	(70%)	2	(11%)	3	(18%)	5	29%
Naso-orbito-ethmoid										
Type I	40		40	(100%)						
Type II	0	(2)		(100%)						
Type III	8	(4)	4	(50%)	4	(50%)			4	50%
Combined	55	(1)	37	(67%)	8	(14%)	10	(18%)	18	(33%)
Total orbital fractures	520	(12)	484	(93%)	23	(4.4%)	13	(2.6%)	36	(7%)

Figure 6.6 (a, b). Mild enophthalmos (submental vertex view) in a patient 1 year after repair of a Type IV orbito-zygomatic fracture. There is mild enophthalmos (2 mm) of the left eye. See Figure 2.2 for CT scans.

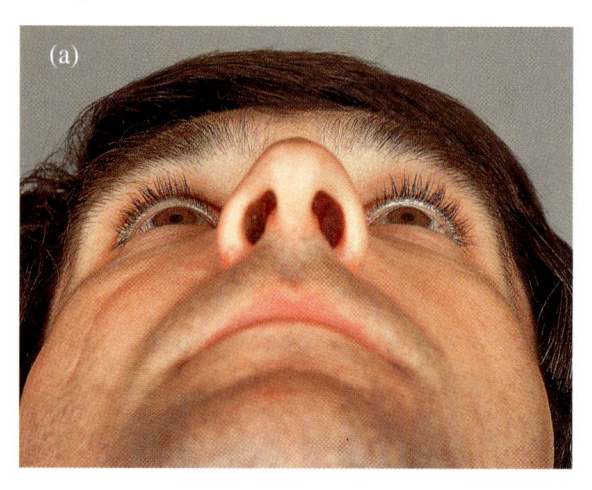

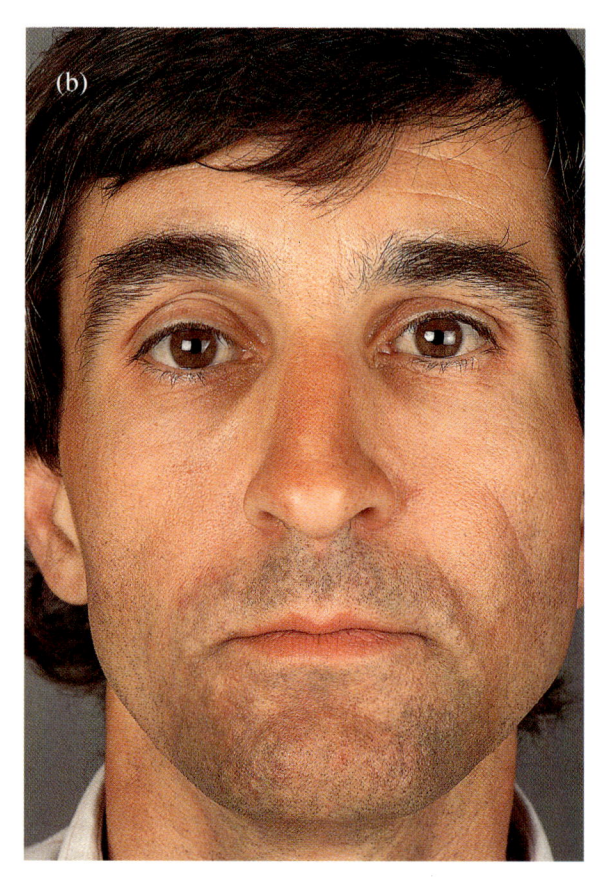

Diplopia

Clinically significant diplopia as a permanent sequel was noted in 13 patients (2.6%) (Table 6.1.17). The underlying mechanisms as well as the importance of an adequate bony reconstruction to prevent adhesions within the orbital connective tissue system were discussed in Chapter 4. The observation that clinically significant diplopia occurred in 5 out of 13 patients with severe enophthalmos underlines the importance of an adequate orbital reconstruction

Significant diplopia also rarely occurred in patients suffering from minor orbital injuries, signifying a neurogenic disorder as the underlying mechanism.

Diplopia in extreme fields of gaze usually does not disturb the patients, though it may be of some hindrance in driving cars or performing certain kinds of sport (ball games).

Revision Surgery

Revision surgery was performed on 83 (18%) patients, the procedures being listed in Table 6.1.18.

Table 6.1.16. Management and outcome in 23 (5%) of 448 patients with visual loss on admission.

Etiology	Therapy	No. patients	Outcome
Globe injury	Enucleation	7	
	Laceration repair	4	
	No therapy	1	
	Total globe injury	12	2 patients recovered to light perception, 10 remained amaurotic
Hematoma/blow-in fracture	Decompression	2	
	Steroids	1	
	Total hematoma/blow-in	3	All 3 patients recovered to full visual acuity
Optic canal fracture	Decompression	1	Visual acuity 0.3
	No therapy	2	Both patients amaurotic
	Total optic canal fracture	3	
Unclear	Decompression	1	Amaurotic
	No therapy	4	1 patient recovered to 0.2 visual acuity
	Total unclear	5	
	Total patients with visual loss	23	

Table 6.1.17. Diplopia in 24 (6%) of 425 patients with orbital fractures (23 amaurotic patients excluded from the total of 448 patients). Significant diplopia is marked in gray.

Degree of enophthalmos	Pat	Normal binocular vision	Mild diplopia[1]	Moderate diplopia[2]	Severe diplopia[3]	Total diplopia
Normal eye position	389	375 (96%)	7 (1.5%)	4 (1%)	3 (1%)	14 (3%)
Mild enophthalmos	23	16 (69%)	5 (21%)	0	0	5 (21%)
Severe enophthalmos	13	6 (46%)	2 (15%)	4 (30%)	1 (7%)	7 (53%)
Total patients	425	401 (94%)	14 (3%)	8 (1.8%)	4 (0.9%)	24 (6%)
Relevant diplopia						12 (3%)

1 = Diplopia in extreme fields of gaze, without significance in daily life, 2 = Diplopia in vertical fields of gaze (disturbing), 3 = Diplopia in straight gaze (extremely disturbing).

Table 6.1.18. Revision surgery in 83 (18.5%) of 448 patients with orbital fractures.

Type of surgery	No. procedures	No. patients	% of 448
Early revisions (<4 weeks)			
Evacuation of hematoma	1	1	
Removal of displaced fragment	2	1	
Closure of oro-antral fistula	2	2	
Total early revisions	5	4	0.8%
Late revisions (>4 weeks)			
Abscess drainage	9	9	
Plate removal	11	5	
Silastic removal	1	1	
Maxillary sinus revision	1	1	
Frontal sinus revision	5	3	
Correction of ectropion	4	3	
Lacrimal duct revision	1	1	
Total late revisions	32	23	5.1%
Secondary corrections			
Scar revisions	31	20	
Removal of palpable/visible plates	22	22	
Major skeletal corrections*	27	12**	
Total secondary corrections	80	56	12.5%
Total revisions	117	83	18.5%

*As described in Chapter 8. **18 patients presented with major skeletal deformities (Table 6.1.14), and corrective surgery was offered to all of them: 4 patients refused further operations, and 2 patients were operated after December 1992. The remaining 12 patients are included in the review of 26 patients with secondary corrections, presented in Section 6.2.

6.2 Review of Patients with Secondary Corrections

Patient Population and Type of Deformities

The review includes 26 from a total of 31 patients, operated on for major posttraumatic deformities between January 1988 and December 1992. Four of these patients were operated on by the author as a consulting doctor in foreign hospitals. Because of incomplete postoperative documentation, however, they were excluded from the review. Another patient was excluded because he left Switzerland 4 weeks after the first reconstructive procedure, making follow-up impossible. The remaining 26 patients were followed up for a minimum of 6 months (mean 13 months, range 6 to 18 months).

Two of the 26 patients had not been treated for their facial fractures at all, 12 patients had their initial surgery at our hospitals (see Table 6.2.1), and 12 had initially been operated on elswhere. There were 18 males and 8 females, with an mean age of 28.5 years (range 19.8 to 61.6 years).

Table 6.2.1. Secondary corrections January 1988 to December 1992.

Number of patients operated on	31*
Excluded	5
Inadequate documentation	4
No follow-up	1
Patients included in review	26

* Three of these patients were operated on by Dr. P. Tessier at the Basel University Hospital. All other patients were operated on by the author.

Enophthalmos was the most often observed deformity, being present in 22 of the 26 patients. Deformities of the inner (telecanthus) and outer orbital frame (flattening of malar eminence) were also frequently present.

A combination of enophthalmos, telecantus, and flattening of the malar eminence was seen in 6 patients. Most of the deformities were unilateral, a bilateral deformity being present in only 5 patients.

The time interval between initial treatment and the first reconstructive procedure varied from 4 weeks to 6 years. In most patients, reconstruction was performed 9 to 15 months after the primary management.

Table 6.2.2. Type of deformities observed in 26 patients (note: most patients presented with more than 1 deformity).

Type of deformity	
Enophthalmos	22
Loss of ocular globe/phtysis	3
Telecanthus/canthal ligament dystopia	14
Malar flattening/increased facial width	12
Supraorbital deformity	3
Total number of deformities observed	54

Table 6.2.3. Time interval between initial treatment and first reconstructive procedure.

Time interval	No. patients
4–8 weeks	2
2–6 months	2
6–12 months	9
1–5 years	10
>5 years	1
No primary repair	2

Operative Treatment

All patients included in this review have been operated on using craniofacial techniques [8, 96, 97] (Table 6.2.4). As reported by other authors, reconstruction usually required several operative procedures [98–100] (Table 6.2.5). All major skeletal corrections were performed during the first operative step, although the nasal osteotomy was repeated in two patients, and deep orbital reconstruction was done repeatedly in 7 patients. In 3 patients, the ini-

Table 6.2.4. Techniques employed during first reconstructive procedure in 26 patients. In several patients, more than one type of reconstructive technique was used.

Reconstructive technique	No.
Osteotomy of zygoma	10
Orbital bone grafting	22
Nasal osteotomy	8
Medial canthopexy without osteotomy	6
Transcranial approach	2
Nasal bone grafts	5
Le Fort I osteotomy	1
Mandibular osteotomy	3

Table 6.2.5. Number of operations per patient.

No. operations per patient	No. patients	No. operations
1 operation	7	7x1 = 7
2 operations	8	8x2 = 16
3 operations	7	7x3 = 21
4 operations	3	3x4 = 12
5 operations	1	1x5 = 5
Total	26	61

tial orbital reconstruction had been combined with osteotomies at the Le Fort I and/or mandibular level. Currently, we prefer to reconstruct the lower face separately.

Solid modelling [101] had been used for 2 patients in order to determine the correct position of the zygoma. This is of some help in analyzing the skeletal deformity, but with advanced experience it can be dispensed with in the planning of posttraumatic corrections.

A total of 61 reconstructive operations were performed on the 26 patients, the number of operations per patient ranging from 1 to 5 (Table 7.2.5).

Results

Follow-up

Clinical and ophthalmological follow-up was obtained with a mean follow-up time of 13 months (range 6 to 18), and every patient was documented with standardized photographs. Postoperative CT scans were done in 13 patients. Esthetic and functional results as well as complications were recorded.

Aesthetic Results

The esthetic results have been classified as "good," "satisfactory," or "unsatisfactory" (Table 6.2.6). Parameters contributing to this rating were the following: overall improvement in light of the initial deformity, degree of enophthalmos correction, and degree of telecanthus correction.[9]

Table 6.2.6. Esthetic results of secondary orbital reconstructions in 26 patients.

Rating	No. of patients	Average no. of operations
Good*	12	1.9 (1 to 3)
Satisfactory**	8	2.2 (1 to 5)
Unsatisfactory	6	2.5 (1 to 4)

* Patients 8.1, 8.2, 8.4, 8.5
** Patient 8.3

The difference between the average number of operations in these groups does not reflect a true tendency. It is merely a reflection of the "escapers" with 4 and 5 surgeries in the latter categories.

Unsatisfactory results arise for various reasons. In 2 patients, complications led to bad results; in a third patient, correction of an enucleated orbit was attempted with temporalis muscle transfer, resulting in an unsightly ptosis. In retrospect, this deformity in retrospect was treated using an unsuitable technique.

A patient with an incorrectly placed orbital meshplate (see Figure 7.27) was not reoperated until 6 months after primary repair, when scarring had already considerably limited ocular motility. A malpositioned graft leading to impaired ocular motility should be replaced as soon as possible!

Scarring may have been responsible for inadequate results in 2 other patients: A fixed deviation of the eye meant that it was questionable whether the correction would be adequate, and the patients had been informed preoperatively about the poor prognosis.

Functional Results: Diplopia

Pre- and postoperative assessment was done in the ophthalmologic clinics of our hospitals (Ophthalmologic Clinic, University Hospital Basel, Switzerland and Eye Hospital Aarau, Switzerland). Eight patients could not be evaluated for binocular vision because of amaurosis or a missing eye. The functional results of the remaining 18 patients are listed in Table 6.2.7.

Table 6.2.7. Binocular vision in 18 patients with posttraumatic deformities (8 of 26 patients excluded for amaurosis or a missing eye).

	Before secondary corr.	After secondary corr.
9 patients	no diplopia	all unchanged
11 patients	diplopia	5 improved
		3 unchanged
		1 worsened

Our functional results parallel the findings of Iliff [102] and contrast with the optimistic reports of several other authors [103, 104, 105]. Diplopia could not be completely eliminated in any of our patients.

However, diplopia in the primary field of vision was eliminated in one patient and the squint angle was reduced in four others. We still recommend bony orbital reconstruction as a first step in diplopia correction, with two important exeptions:
– Minimal enophthalmos without obvious orbital wall defects,
– Severely limited ocular motility with diplopia in all fields except in the primary field of vision. In these patients, secondary correction may induce diplopia in the primary field of gaze.

Complications

Five patients (15%) presented with complications requiring operative treatment (Table 6.2.8). Two patients presented with an orbital abscess requiring surgical drainage. Both patients had suffered from a cold a few days previously. The abscess was localized in the upper medial quadrant of the orbit, indicating that it had entered through the frontal sinus. As in primary repair, infectious complications mainly originated in the frontal sinus, whereas problems with the maxillary sinus were not observed. The data underline the importance of adequate frontal sinus management.

Two patients suffered from severe ocular complications. In one patient, direct optic nerve injury occurred because of a dislocated bone graft (Figure 6.6). The graft was removed, but the patient's injured eye remained blind. A second patient developed an endophthalmitis after ptosis correction, resulting in loss of the eye, which had already been amaurotic since the accident.

One overcontoured nasal bone graft perforated the skin. After reduction of the graft with a rongeur, uneventful healing took place. No extrusion of nasal grafts as reported by Cohen [98] occurred.

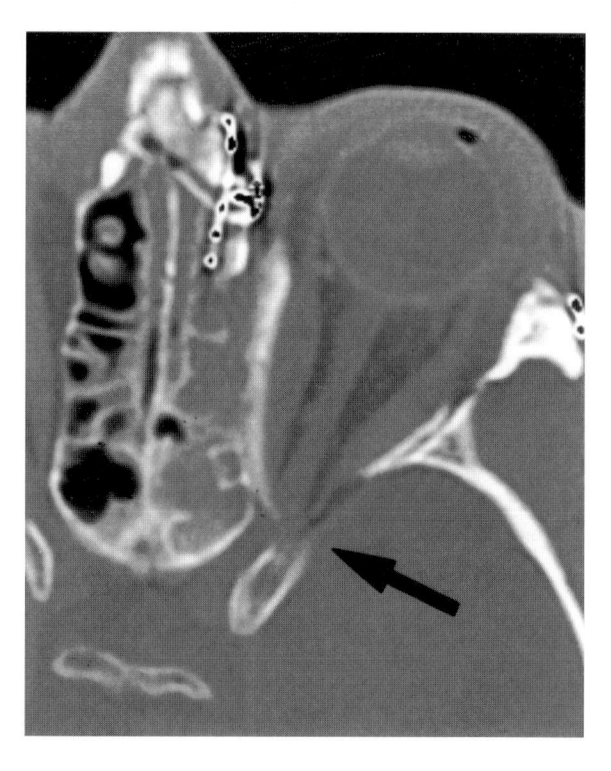

Figure 6.6. Direct injury to the optic nerve by a displaced bone graft. During secondary orbital reconstruction, a bone graft was placed too far posteriorly, resulting in direct injury to the optic nerve. Despite operative revision, the patient lost his vision in this eye.

Table 6.2.8. Complications of secondary corrections in 5 (15%) of 26 patients with 59 reconstructive procedures.

Type of complication	No. of patients	Treatment
Orbital abcess	2	1 drainage
		1 drainage + obliteration of frontal sinus
Exposure of nasal bone graft	1	Contouring
Optic nerve damage	1	Decompression (not successful)
Endophthalmitis after ptosis surgery	1	Enucleation of affected eye

Chapter 7
Operative Management of Orbital Fractures

Because of the wide spectrum of orbital fractures, operative treatment necessarily includes a variety of procedures, ranging from closed reduction to complex orbital reconstruction making extensive use of craniofacial techniques.

As already mentioned (Chapter 4), fractures may involve parts or the whole of the orbital frame, the orbital walls, or both. Technical questions regarding repair of these different parts of the orbit are dealt with in individual sections of this chapter.

7.1 Basic Principles

Exposure

The type and extent of exposure depends on the localization and pattern of the orbital injury as well as on the presence of associated midfacial fractures. Local incisions are used for nonfragmented orbito-zygomatic fractures and for defects in the anterior and middle part of the orbital floor. Naso-ethmoid fractures, complex orbito-zygomatic fractures, and defects in the posterior third of the orbit require wide exposure via combined local and coronal approaches.

Lower Eyelid Approach

The lower eyelid approach provides access to the infraorbital rim and orbital floor. Several types of incisions are described, either through the conjunctiva [106] or transcutaneously, each individual type having advantages and disadvantages [107, 108].

Our preferred cutaneous incisions are the subciliary incision and the mid-lower eyelid incision.

The latter is used in most cases. It combines a virtually invisible scar with a low incidence of complications [107]. The incision starts medially about 3 mm below the lid margin and is directed latero-caudally (Figure 7.1, right eye). To avoid a visible scar, it should not extend laterally more than two-thirds of the lid, so that access to the lateral orbital wall is limited. The incision is combined with either a upper blepharoplasty incision or a coronal incision.

In selected cases, a subciliary incision is used (Figure 7.1, left eye). It is placed 2–3 mm caudal to the lid margin and can be extended beyond the lateral canthus, providing generous exposure of the orbital ring up to the zygomatico-frontal suture as well as to the orbital floor and lateral orbital wall. This enables exposure of the whole anterior orbit with a single approach [109]. The main disadvantage of this incision is the relative frequency of lid shortening and scleral show [110]. Our experience has shown that this complication is likely to occur especially in older patients with lid laxity, and in patients with thin lids and hypoplastic orbicularis oculi muscles: In these patients, a mid-lower eyelid inci-

Figure 7.1. Anterior orbital approach. On the left eyelid, a subciliary incision is outlined, running 2–3 mm below the lid margin. It can be extended beyond the lateral canthus, thereby providing exposure of the anterior orbit with a single approach. Contraindications are lid laxity, a hypoplastic orbicularis oculi muscle, and prior lid incisions. In these cases, the mid-lower eyelid incision, outlined on the right eyelid, is employed. To avoid a visible scar, the incision should not extend laterally beyond the corneal limbus. Access to the fronto-zygomatic suture is obtained with an additional upper blepharoplasty incision.

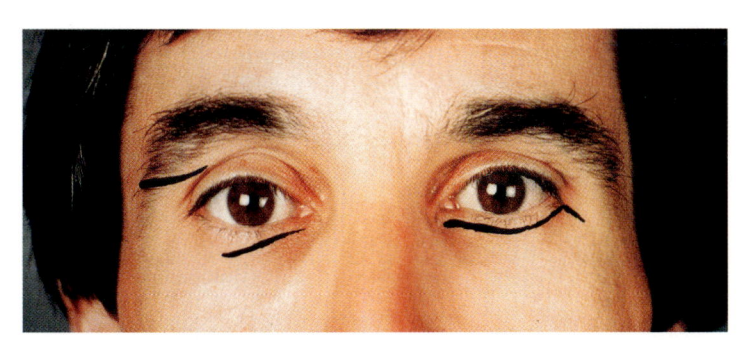

sion should be used. The subciliary incision should also be avoided in secondary corrections, since pre-existing lid problems are likely to be increased by this approach (see Chapter 8).

Both of these incisions are designed as a skin-muscle flap. The dissection must be carried precisely along the orbicularis oculi muscle and not along the orbital septum (Figure 7.2, skin muscle flap), as damage to this structure is likely to result in lid shortening. If the subciliary incision is used, a cuff of orbicularis oculi muscle must be left attached to the lid margin.

Upper Blepharoplasty Incision

The upper blepharoplasty incision provides exposure of the fronto-zygomatic suture and to a limited extent of the lateral orbital wall. It is used in combination with a mid-lower eyelid incision (Figure 7.1).

An incision is created in the skin of one of the upper lid folds, which is continued through the periosteum along the lateral orbital rim, the result of which is a 70° change in the orientation of the wound.

Intraoral Approach

The upper buccal sulcus incision provides exposure of the zygomatico-maxillary buttress, which is one of the most reliable points for reduction and fixation of the zygoma. This incision may be combined with anterior orbital and with coronal approaches.

In patients who wear dentures, this incision is better placed on the alveolar crest to avoid scar formation in the buccal sulcus, which could interfere with denture wear. A vertical backcut in the incisor area can permit tension-free elevation of the mucosal flap.

Coronal Incision

The coronal incision exposes the entire upper mid-face skeleton including the zygomatic arches. It provides three-dimensional visualization of the orbital frame, and exposes the medial and lateral orbital wall as well as the orbital roof. It is therefore the approach of choice for complex orbito-zygomatic and nasoethmoid fractures as well as for all injuries involving the posterior third of the internal orbit.

For preparation, a 1-cm wide strip of hair is shaved, allowing for a straight incision from ear to

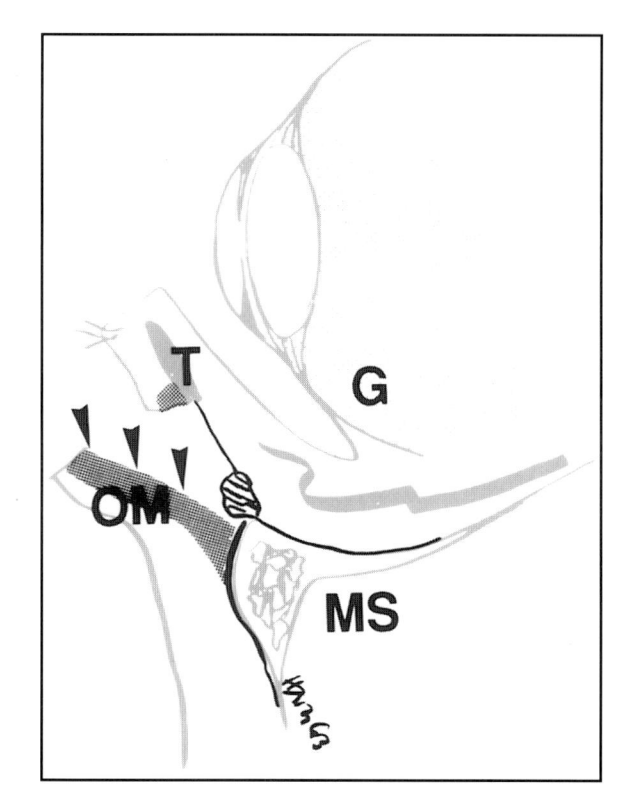

Figure 7.2. Lower eyelid approach. A muscle splitting incision is employed. Damage to the orbital septum is avoided by dissecting strictly on the posterior surface of the orbicularis oculi muscle (arrows). The preseptal fat pad (removed during lower lid blepharoplasty) is left attached to the septum. G: ocular globe. T: tarsal plate. OM: orbicularis oculi muscle. MS: maxillary sinus.

ear. Infiltration with a local anesthetic containing a vasoconstrictor considerably reduces bleeding.

When the dissection is carried down to the zygomatic arch, care must be taken to avoid injury to the frontal branch of the facial nerve. This branch crosses the zygomatic arch about 2 cm anterior to the external auditory meatus, travelling superiorly into the frontal area [111]; it is therefore included in the flap. Injury to this nerve is safely avoided by approaching the zygomatic arch in the superficial temporal fat pad [95], thereby leaving a sturdy fascia medial to the nerve (Figures 7.3, 7.4, 7.5).

No attempt should be made to expose the orbit through a so-called hemi-coronal flap. The exposure will always be inadequate, especially in the nasoethmoid region.

Marginotomies

Visibility and access to the posterior orbit can be enhanced with marginotomies [97]. The inferior

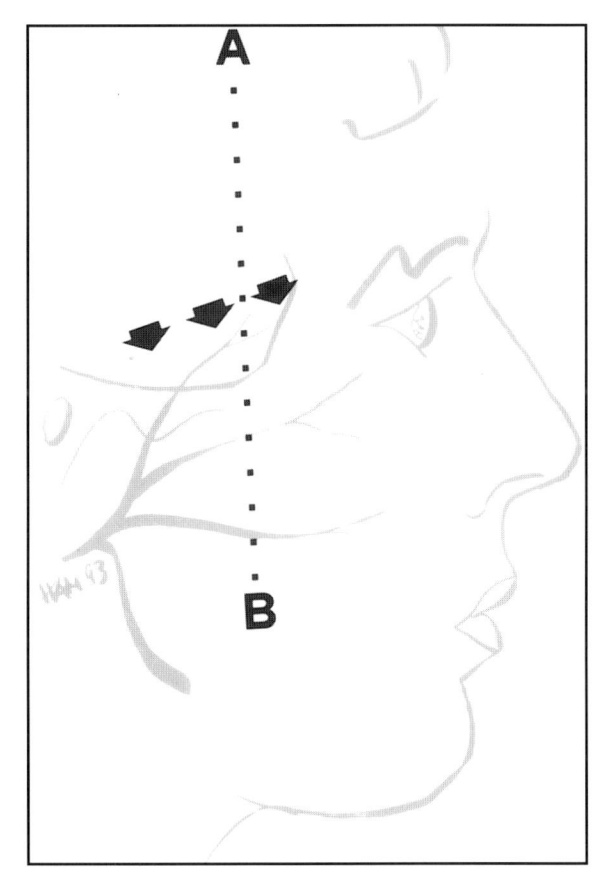

Figure 7.3. Coronal approach. The frontal branch of the facial nerve crosses the zygomatic arch 2 cm anterior to the external auditory meatus. If access to the arch is necessary, the nerve is protected by including it into the flap. The arrows indicate the line of entry into the fat pad. The dotted line between A and B indicates the plane of cross-section, shown in Figure 7.4.

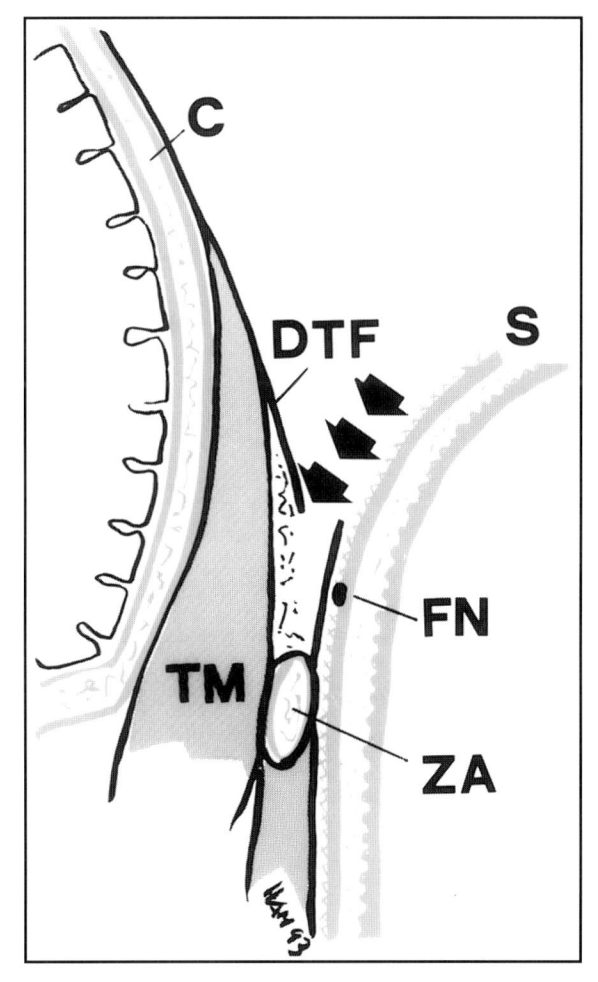

Figure 7.4. About 4 cm above the zygomatic arch, the deep temporal fascia is incised (arrows) and the dissection is continued within the temporal fat pad. C: calvaria. S: scalp flap. DTF: deep temporal fascia. TM: temporalis muscle. FN: frontal nerve. ZA: zygomatic arch.

marginotomy is rarely indicated in primary fracture repair, while superior marginotomies are often utilized (Case 7.3, Figure 7.25).

The superior marginotomy removes the superomedial portion of the orbital ring, which is simultaneously part of the anterior wall of the frontal sinus (Figure 7.6). Temporary removal permits access to the fronto-ethmoid transition and the anterior cranial base, facilitating subcranial inspection of the skull base and duraplasty [112], when necessary.

Following the medial orbital wall, the optic foramen is easily exposed by this route, allowing for optic canal decompression.

Rigid Fixation

Rigid fixation with plates and screws has become the foundation for modern fracture treatment, with many advantages compared to wire fixation. Whereas interosseous wires are capable of resisting only tensile forces, rigid plates provide torsional and buttressing stability and additionally allow the bridging of discontinuities and fragmentation. In many instances, plates are easier to handle than wires. For example, passing a wire back and forth can be a tedious procedure, whereas screw insertion is unidirectional.

The different hardware systems on the market are all based on the principle of adaptation osteosynthesis with self-tapping screws [113–116]. The plates are aligned along the midfacial or orbital frame butresses in order to reestablish the normal loadpath [117]. They may also be used to stabilize bone grafts.

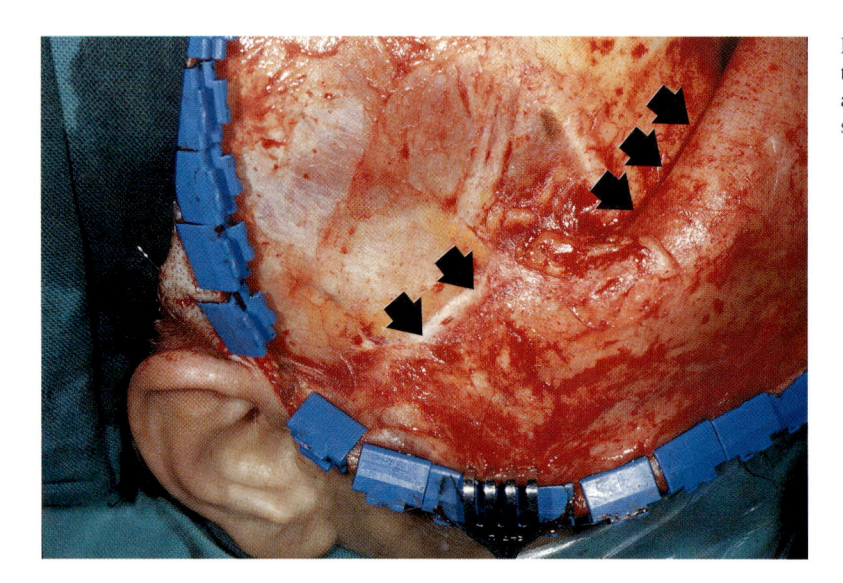

Figure 7.5. Coronal approach. Incision of the deep temporal fascia (arrows center; arrows upper right indicate position of the supraorbital rim).

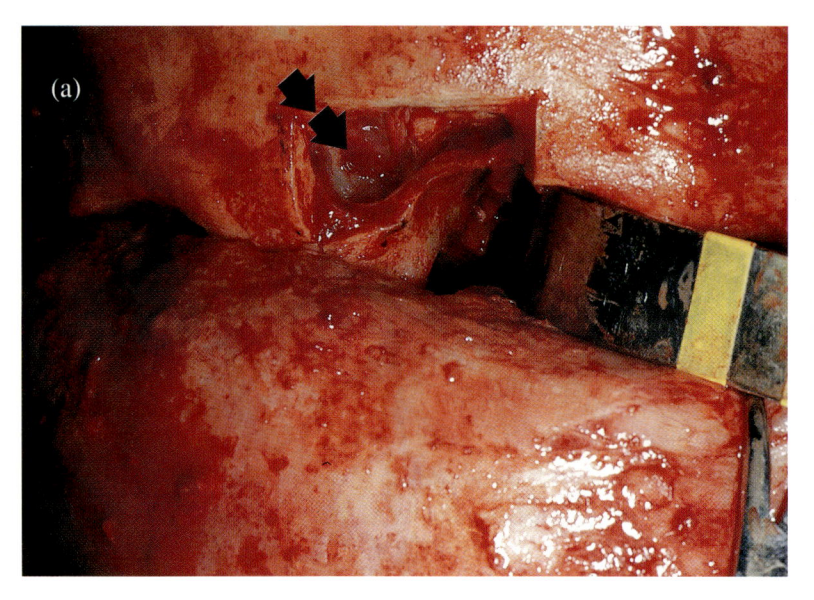

Figure 7.6 (a, b). Intraoperative view (a) and schematic drawing (b) of a superior marginotomy. The malleable retractor is inserted into the left orbit. The marginotomy fragment has been removed, exposing the transition between the anterior part of the orbital roof (which is also the floor of the frontal sinus) and the medial wall (arrows in (a)). Removal of this bone with a rongeur provides generous exposure of the frontoethmoidal transition and the upper part of the medial orbital wall back to the optic canal. CF: coronal flap. MR: malleable retractor.

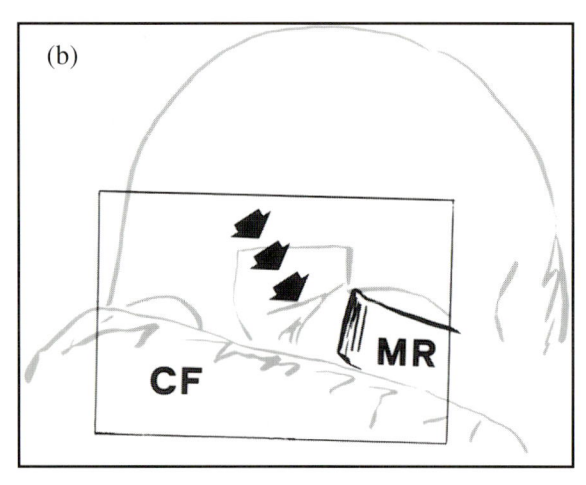

Most systems include miniplates and microplates, such as the AO craniofacial system (Synthes [USA], Mathys and Stratec [Switzerland]), which we use. The AO craniofacial set provides screws with a diameter of 1.5 and 2.0 mm for the minisystem, and 1 mm screws for the microsystem [118].

Titanium is the preferred implant material, because it is presently considered to be the most biocompatible material for metallic implants [119, 120]. According to the current opinion, implants made of titanium may be permanently left in situ. A particular advantage of titanium is the avoidance of interference with MRI imaging and the lack of CT-scan scattering effects [121].

Bone Graft Harvesting of the Calvarium

Bone grafts are the material of choice for the reconstruction of large orbital wall defects [110, 122]. The calvaria has become the most important donor site, as it has the advantage of being available in the same operative field as the reconstruction [96]. Its low resorption rate, especially when rigidly fixed [123], further speaks in favor of this source.

Depending on needs, the grafts may be harvested as small chips or as rectangular pieces. If the periosteum is left attached to the bone, a flexible compound of bone and periosteum can be harvested [124].

To obtain rectangular pieces of outer table, the left or right temporo-parietal area is exposed and the shape of the graft is outlined with a burr or a saw (Figure 7.7). Harvesting is performed with a chisel [125]. The mean bone thickness in the frontoparietal area is about 7 mm [126], which allows for harvesting a stable 2 mm thick graft. Fracturing of the brittle bone is avoided by exactly dividing the bone in the diploic layer.

Accidental full thickness harvesting is reported to occur in up to 14.5% of cases [127], our own rate being around 12%, with a single case of dural laceration occurring without any sequelae (unpublished data). However, serious complications are reported [128], and cranial bone graft harvesting remains a procedure to be performed with great deliberation.

Repositioning of Soft Tissues with Suspension Sutures

Repair of complex fractures requires extensive detachment of the associated soft tissues, with undermining of the entire hemiface in the subperiosteal plane often necessary to gain adequate exposure and mobilization of fragments for reduction. Without repositioning, these soft tissue structures heal in a ptotic position, creating the impression of inadequate malar prominence (Figure 7.8 b). Loss of soft tissue support can cause eyelid shortening.

To prevent this, the soft tissues of the anterior and lateral cheek are superiorly resuspended with heavy sutures, anchored at the infraorbital rim and the temporal fascia [129] (Figure 7.8 a). Currently, we also reattach the upper eyebrow to the supraorbital rim to avoid malpositioning, which has been observed in several patients.

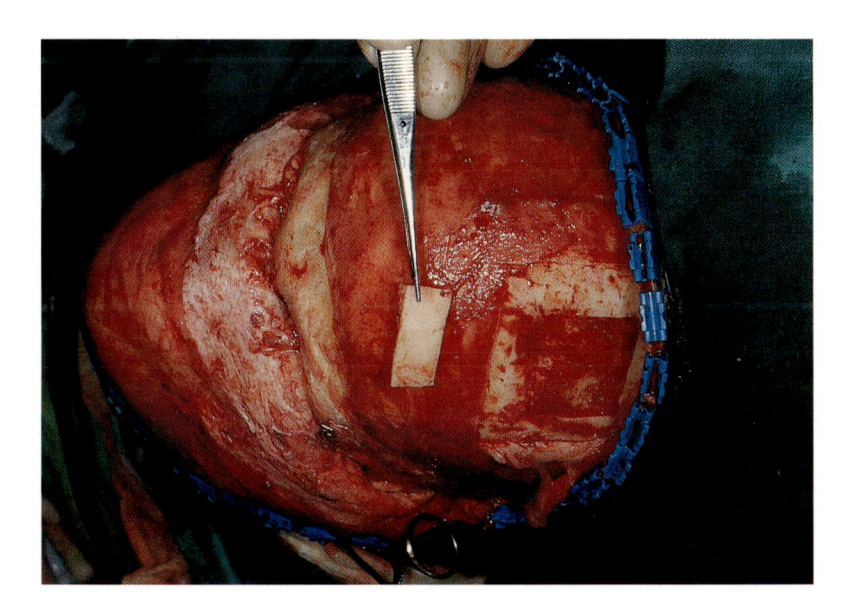

Figure 7.7. Harvesting of outer table bone grafts. Rectangular pieces 2 x 3 cm are outlined with a burr or a saw in the temporo-parietal region. Removal is performed with a chisel.

Reinsertion of the lateral canthal ligament is also part of the soft tissue resuspension, although this ligament cannot be identified as a distinct anatomic structure. The procedure is performed by passing a 2.0 suture through the deep tissue in the area of the lateral angle of the eyelid and then fixing it to the inner aspect of the lateral orbital rim via osseous burrholes in a slightly overcorrected position.

7.2 Orbito-Zygomatic Fractures (Outer Orbital Frame)

Nonfragmented Orbito-Zygomatic Fractures

Isolated Orbito-Zygomatic Fractures

Isolated orbito-zygomatic fractures are the most common injuries involving the orbit, usually from low-velocity trauma.

The zygoma may be nondisplaced and minimally or highly displaced. Depending on the level of displacement, the changes in orbital volume may be mild, moderate, or extensive. Associated defects in the orbital floor requiring bridging are observed in about half of the orbito-zygomatic fractures. Al-

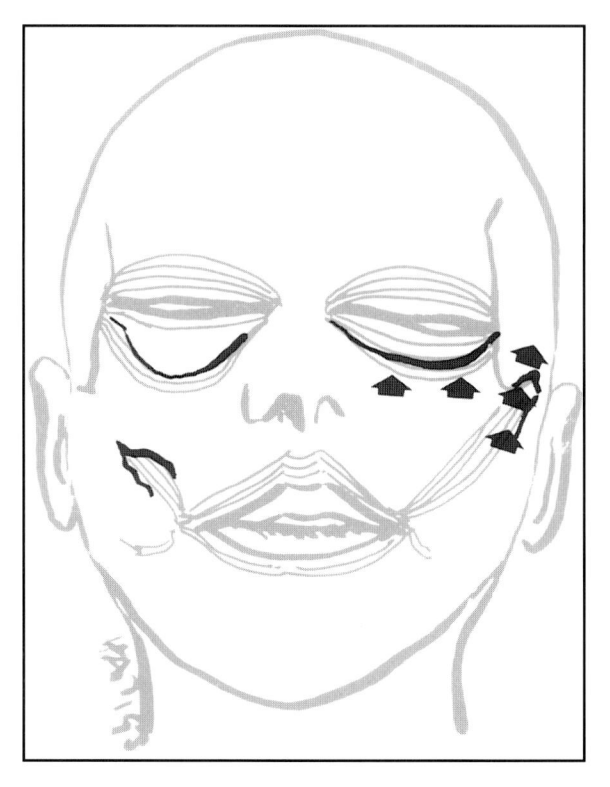

Figure 7.8 (a). Resuspension of soft tissues. Right hemiface: During subperiosteal exposure of fractures, the insertions of facial muscles are released. Left hemiface: Displacement of these insertions is corrected with anchoring sutures according to subperiosteal face-lift techniques.

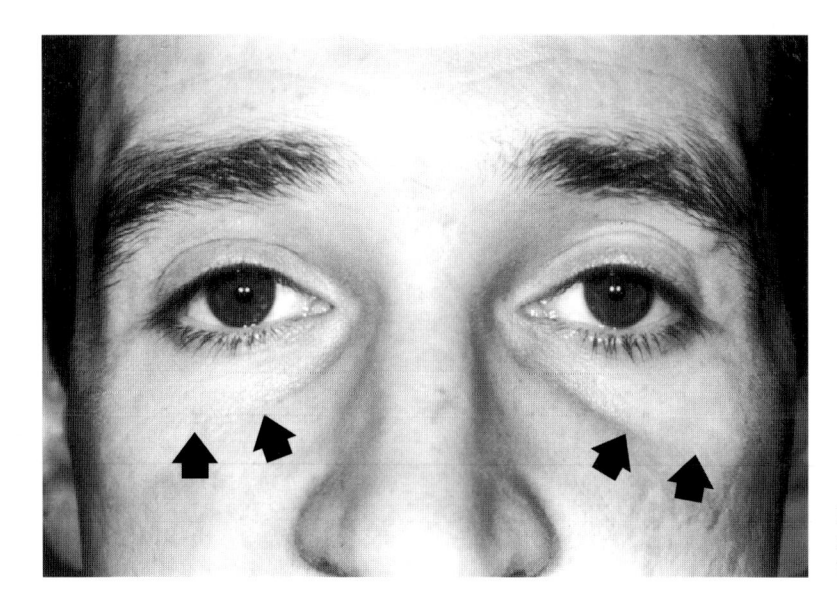

Figure 7.8 (b). Soft tissue sagging (arrows) after repair of bilateral orbital fractures without soft tissue resuspension.

though these fractures are classified as nonfragmented (Chapter 3), an isolated fragment at the infraorbital rim or some degree of fragmentation at the zygomatico-maxillary buttress is often present, making open reduction and fixation necessary.

Principles of Management
The literature is replete with data about the management of orbitozygomatic fractures [130–135], with considerable differences in treatment recommendations. Rohrich et al. [136] summarized the findings as follows:
– There is a subset of orbitozygomatic fractures that can be managed with closed reduction. This includes nonfragmented fractures that are stable postreduction.
– Other orbitozygomatic fractures require open reduction and internal fixation
– Of the numerous methods available, miniplate and/or microplate fixation seem to provide the best results with the lowest complication rates.

Number of Plates
Stabilization with a minimum of two plates is recommended. This recommendation is supported by theoretical [117], experimental [133, 137] and clinical data [135, 138, 139]. The two plates are placed either along the infraorbital and lateral orbital margin (Figure 7.9) or along the infraorbital margin and the zygomatico-maxillary buttress.

Surgical Technique
Closed reduction can be accomplished with a J-shaped hook inserted transcutaneously, the tip engaging the undersurface of the zygomatic body to allow for outward and forward traction. The index finger of the left hand palpates the infraorbital rim or the zygomatico-maxillary buttress to assess reduction. After reduction has been achieved, stability is checked by moderately pressing the zygomatic body inwards.

If open reduction is necessary, an intraoral approach is combined with an anterior orbital approach (subciliary or mid-lower eyelid/blepharoplasty). The most important landmark for reduction is the lateral orbital wall, where the zygoma has a long articulation with the greater sphenoid wing (sphenozygo-

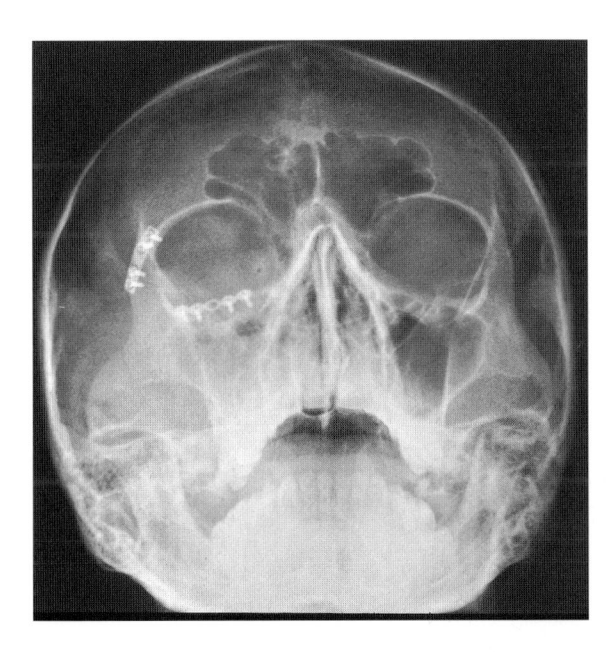

Figure 7.9. Stabilization of a simple orbito-zygomatic fracture with two miniplates provides adequate stability. Alternatively, the plates could be placed along the zygomatico-maxillary buttress and the infraorbital rim.

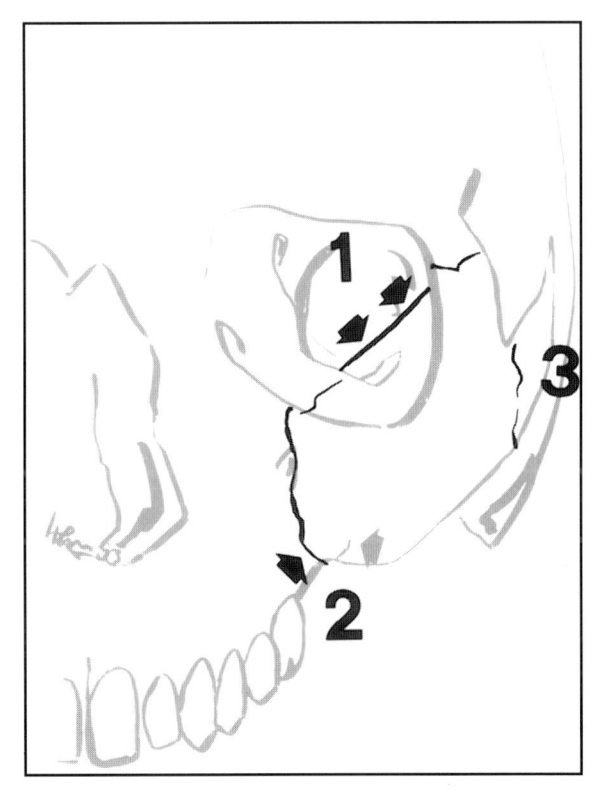

Figure 7.10. Landmarks for reduction of the zygomatic body. The lateral orbital wall (1) with its long articulation between the zygomatic body and the greater sphenoid wing is the most important site for alignment and should be exposed during every open reduction. The zygomatico-maxillary buttress (2) provides a second reliable site of reduction. In cases with severe fragmentation of this area, or if an associated Le Fort I fracture makes this buttress unreliable, the zygomatic arch (3) must be exposed and utilized. If the zygomatic body itself is fragmented, all three sites of reduction need to be be exposed.

matic suture, Figure 7.10). The zygomatico-maxillary buttress is used as a second landmark. If there is extensive fragmentation of this buttress, or if an associated Le Fort I fracture renders it unreliable, the zygomatic arch is used as an additional reduction and stabilization point [140, 141].

Routine exploration of the orbital floor after reduction of displaced orbito-zygomatic fractures is recommended to avoid undetected incarceration of periorbital tissue between bone fragments in the orbital floor during the reduction maneuver.

Orbito-Zygomatic Fracture as Part of a Complex Midface or Panfacial Fracture

If a zygomatic fracture (fragmented or nonfragmented) is part of a midfacial or panfacial fracture, the zygoma becomes an important buttress securing the correct antero-posterior position of the maxilla and eventually the nasal bones.

Reduction of the maxilla and the nasal bones (inner facial or orbital frame) depends on the accurate position of the zygomatic body, which is therefore a key element and utilized as the first step of the multiple fracture repair [6]. Because the only reliable landmarks for its correct positioning are the zygomatic arch and the lateral orbital wall [140], a complete exposure with combined anterior and coronal approach is necessary. Technical details are described below.

Fragmented Orbito-Zygomatic Fractures

These fractures often result from a direct high-velocity injury [1]. The zygomatic body and/or arch is fractured in multiple segments (Figure 7.11). There is loss of anterior projection of the zygomatic body, usually combined with increased facial width. Complex orbital wall defects may or may not be present. In these injuries, correct antero-posterior reduction and stabilization are achieved with the zygomatic arch as a guiding buttress [140, 141] (Figure 7.12).

Exposure is obtained with a combined anterior and coronal approach. Often, soft-tissue contracture causes secondary dislocation of fragments, which are difficult to align. For this reason, extensive elevation of periosteum and freeing of the masseter muscle insertion is indicated.

The zygomatic arch is exposed posteriorly to the temporal bone, where an oblique fracture with backward shearing and thus shortening of the arch is frequently found (Case 7.1).

Stabilization is initiated with insertion of a temporary wire at the fronto-zygomatic suture, and as the next step, the arch is reconstructed. If a fracture at the root is present, a lag screw or a short plate is now placed. The rest of the arch is reconstructed with one plate, which usually does not need bending.

After reconstruction of the arch, the fractures of the zygomatic body are addressed (No. 2 in Figure 7.12). Correct alignment of the fragments along the lateral orbital wall must be checked before stabilization with plates. If the zygomatico-maxillary but-

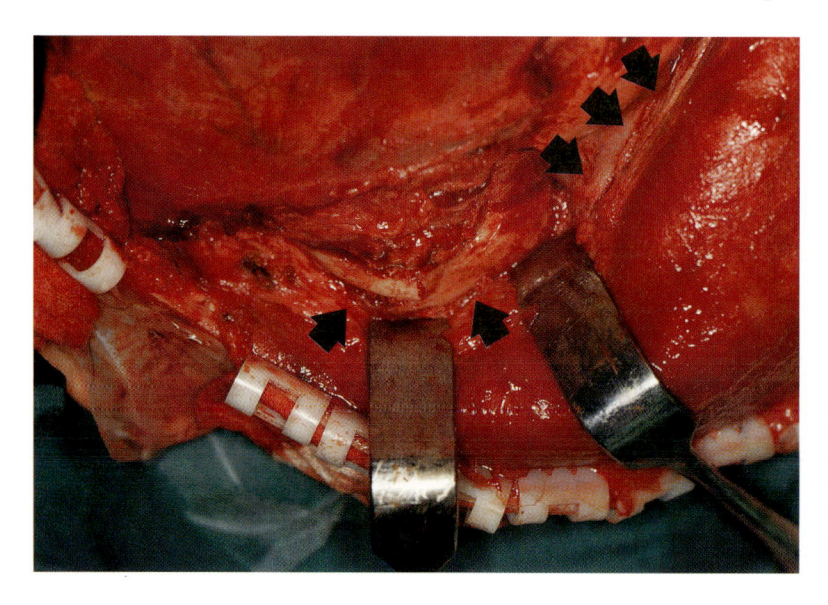

Figure 7.11. Fragmented orbito-zygomatic fracture. There is loss of malar projection and increased facial width due to outward bending of the arch. Arrows center: fragmented and shortened zygomatic arch. Arrows upper right: supraorbital margin.

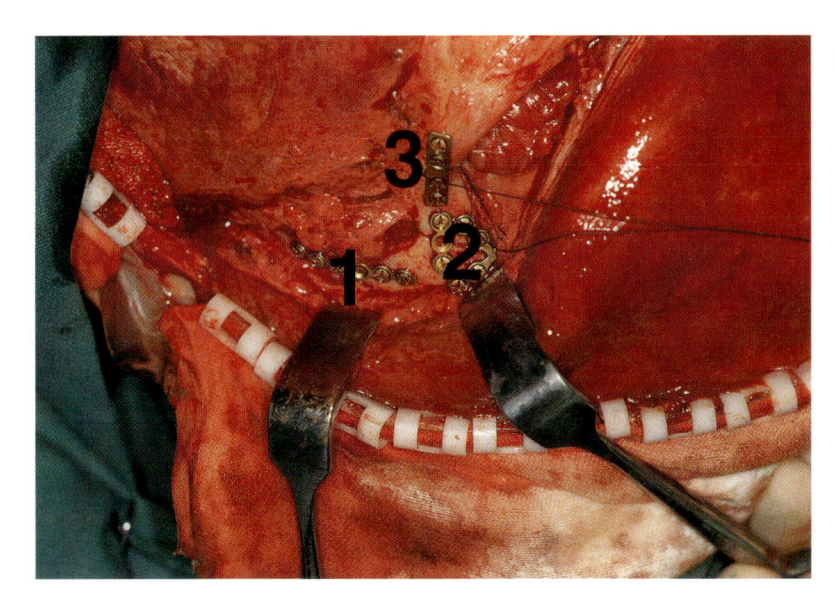

Figure 7.12. Stabilization of a fragmented orbito-zygomatic fracture. After reconstruction of the zygomatic arch (1), the body of the zygoma is plated (2). Finally, the temporary wire at the fronto-zygomatic suture is replaced with a plate (3).

tress is intact, it is used as an additional landmark. Finally, the wire at the zygomatico-frontal suture is replaced by a plate.

The zygomatico-maxillary buttress often shows a minor degree of fragmentation. Bony defects of the buttress itself or of the maxillary sinus walls can be reconstructed with outer table calvarial grafts.

Rigid fixation of the infraorbital rim is performed last. If the nasal bones are stable, a microplate may be used to adapt small bone fragments. As soon as the inner orbital frame is involved, the mechanical load is greater and a stronger plate is necessary.

Fragmented orbitozygomatic fractures are always associated with some degree of orbital-wall defect, which has to be repaired after stabilization of the orbital frame. These problems are adressed in Section 7.4.

7.3 Naso-Orbito-Ethmoid Fractures (Inner Orbital Frame)

Treatment of naso-orbito-ethmoid (NOE) fractures involves reconstruction of the complex three-dimensional anatomy of the glabellar region and often the management of associated nasal, frontal sinus, and skull-base injuries. Operative treatment, consisting of an extended open approach with anatomic reduction and rigid fixation of bone fragments, should be undertaken as early as possible. Management of the medial canthal tendon or a tendon attached to the bone fragment requires special attention.

Exposure is achieved with a coronal flap. Local incisions have the combined disadvantage of a visible scar and limited access. In virtually all cases, additional lower eyelid and intraoral incisions are necessary.

Stabilization of naso-orbito-ethmoid fractures is achieved with mini- and microplates. The microplates are helpful in aligning the very small fragments of the nasal root together, and they may also be used to link a large central fragment to the frontal bone. Miniplates are indicated when increased mechanical stability is required. Because of their relative thickness, however, miniplates should not be employed anterior to the lacrimal crest. In addition, transnasal wires are utilized to secure the central bone fragment against outward rotation and for direct canthopexy (see below).

Management of the Central Fragment

The basic problem in NOE fracture treatment lies in managing the central fragment bearing the canthal ligament [29] Typical fracture patterns and their identification are described in Chapter 3. The type of reconstruction depends on the position, degree of fragmentation, and soft-tissue attachments of the central fragment:
- In typeI injuries, there is a large canthal-ligament-bearing fragment that may be reduced and stabilized with plates alone (Figure 7.13). Here, a mini-

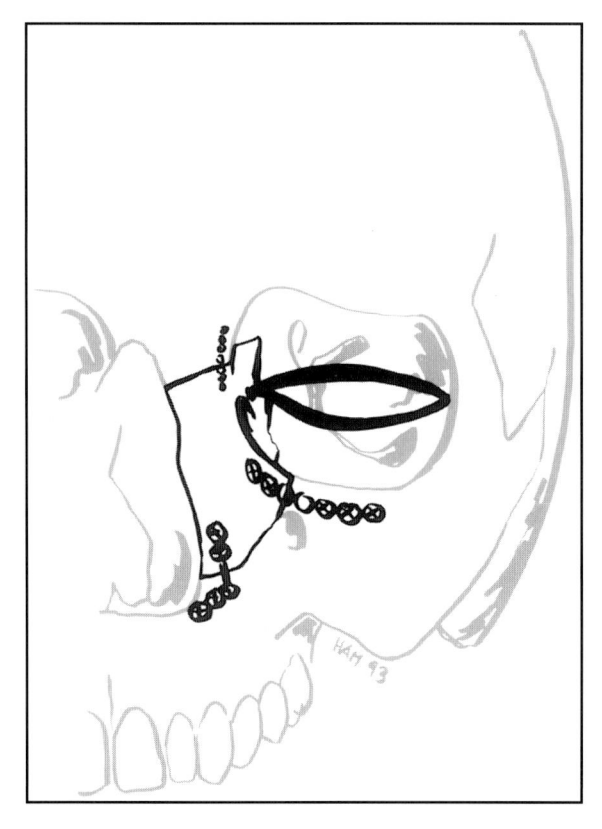

Figure 7.13. Stabilization of a naso-orbito-ethmoidal fracture type I. The central fragment can be adequately stabilized against outward rotation with plate fixation.

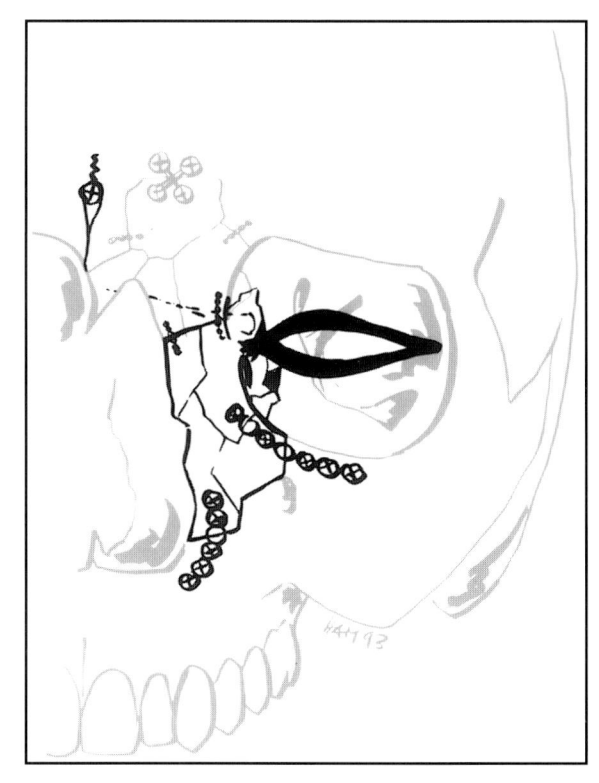

Figure 7.14. Stabilization of a naso-orbito-ethmoidal fracture type II. In addition to plate fixation, a transnasal wire is inserted which stabilizes the fragment against outward rotation. The wire must be placed posterior to the lacrimal crest.

plate at the infraorbital rim is used to stabilize the fragment, as a microplate would be insufficient to stabilize the fragment against rotation. Before placing the plate at the infraorbital rim, one must verify the articulation of the fragment with the nasal process of the frontal bone in order to avoid malrotation. This fracture site may be stabilized with a microplate.
- In type II injuries, the fragmented inner orbital frame is reconstructed using microplates. In order to avoid outward rotation of the fragment bearing the canthal ligament, stabilization is performed with a transnasal wire inserted posterior to the lacrimal crest (Figure 7.14). Thus, the correct rotational position of the central fragment is ensured and widening of the nasal root avoided.
- In type III injuries, the central fragment is too small to be utilized for canthopexy. There can be avulsion of the medial canthal ligament, although this is an uncommon finding. Reconstruction of these fractures requires a direct transnasal canthopexy.

Initially, the canthal ligament is completely detached, because if a bone fragment is left attached to the canthal ligament, it can interfere with direct canthopexy. The small fragments of the inner orbital frame are now aligned and stabilized with microplates.

Transnasal canthopexy is the most difficult part of the procedure and involves two steps. Initially, the ligament is identified and held with a suture, something easily performed through a small transverse incision medial to the palpebral fissure [142]. This suture is linked to the transnasal wire.

The second step lies in electing the insertion point of the transnasal wire, which should be inserted posteriorly and superiorly to the lacrimal fossa. In most cases, however, the fragile bone of this area is fragmented, so that the insertion point of the transnasal wire has to be constructed, either by drilling a hole through a bone graft inserted along the medial wall or with the help of a miniplate [143] (Figure 7.15).

Tightening the transnasal cantopexy is not done until the bone graft reconstruction of the internal orbit has been completed, as the insertion of bone grafts

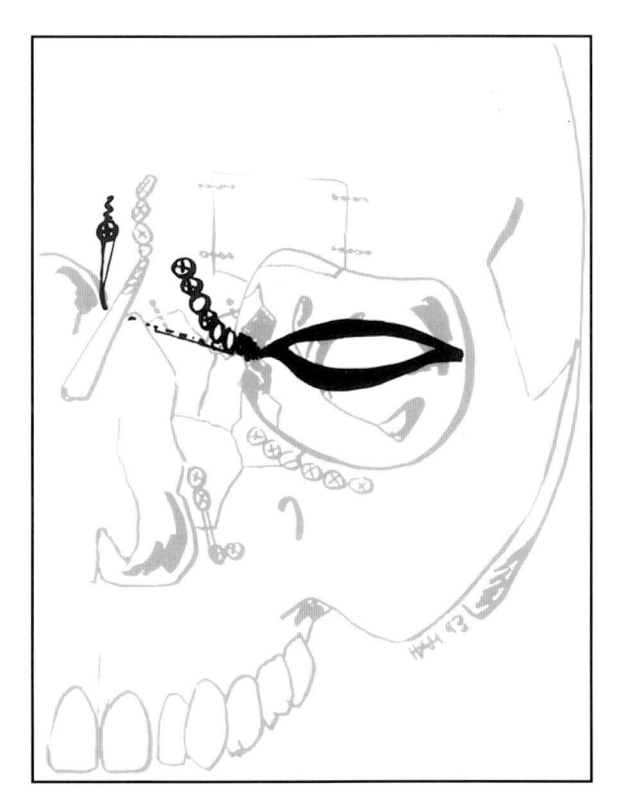

Figure 7.15. Stabilization of a naso-orbito-ethmoidal fracture type III. A sizable central fragment cannot be identified, making direct transnasal canthopexy necessary. The insertion point is created with the help of a miniplate. Subcranial exploration of the anterior skull base, when indicated, may be performed via a superior marginotomy.

for the medial wall is facilitated by free canthal ligaments.

Nasal Reconstruction

Naso-orbito-ethmoid fractures are always associated with nasal trauma. Often the bony and cartilagineous septae are fragmented with a resultant collapsed and shortened nose.

If there is a lack of septal support, dorsal bone grafting is necessary to reestablish the height and anterior projection of the nose [144, 145], cranial bone grafts being the first choice [146]. The graft serves as a cantilever onto which the nasal septum, together with the attached upper lateral cartilages, is resuspended. The tip of the graft is placed between the domes of the lower lateral cartilages in order to obtain a smooth contour.

For precise graft placement, an open rhinoplasty approach is preferred.

Naso-Orbito-Ethmoid Fracture-Related Problems

Lacrimal Duct Injuries

Although the lacrimal apparatus has an intimate relationship to the medial canthal tendon, injury resulting in its obstruction or disruption is rarely encountered. Primary exploration of the lacrimal apparatus is therefore not recommended unless an open laceration is present. In these cases, fine silicone tubes may be utilized to support the canaliculi.

Frontal Sinus and Anterior Cranial Base Injuries

A high percentage of naso-orbito-ethmoid injuries are associated with fractures of the frontal sinus and/or the anterior cranial base with cerebro-spinal fluid (CSF) leakage. In these cases, reconstruction is combined with frontal sinus exploration and repair, and can include subcranial exploration of the anterior skull base [112].

The management of frontal sinus injuries depends upon the level of injury as well as on the anatomic situation, i.e. the size and shape of the frontal sinus. Our own management protocol essentially follows the guidelines published by Stanley [147]:
- Reconstruction is the first option, performed in all injuries limited to the anterior wall as well as in nondisplaced or minimally displaced posterior wall fractures.
- Fractures involving the frontonasal duct constitute an indication for complete removal of the sinus mucosa and obliteration of the sinus, our preferred materials being fascia or fat. A wide fronto-ethmoidal transition, however, may preclude obliteration of the sinus, because an inferior closure cannot be obtained.
- Cranialization is rarely indicated; the only injuries that require it are fragmented fractures of the posterior wall. Cranialization is preferably avoided in order to keep potential sinus complications extracranial.

Sequence of Operative Steps in Repair of Naso-Orbito-Ethmoidal Fractures

- Following exposure, as a first step the posterior table of the frontal sinus and anterior cranial base

is explored and repaired where indicated. Access is obtained either by removing the fragments of an anterior wall fracture or with a superior marginotomy.
- The transnasal wires reducing the central fragment and/or the wires for direct transnasal canthopexy are placed. Bone fragments are reduced, but the direct canthopexy wires are not yet tightened.
- Bone graft reconstruction of the orbits is now performed as necessary.
- As the next step, the anterior frontal sinus wall is reconstructed and the fronal sinus can be obliterated.
- Finally, the canthopexy wires are tightened.

7.4 Fractures of the Internal Orbit

Fractures and defects of the internal orbit may occur as isolated injuries or associated with fractures of the orbital frame. In the majority of cases, the injuries are confined to the orbital floor and are defined as blow-out fractures[10]. Isolated fractures of the medial wall or the roof are less common and in most cases result from direct trauma to the overlying structures of the orbital frame. The lateral orbital wall, which is usually involved in low-energy orbito-zygomatic fractures, is rarely defective following correct three-dimensional reduction of the zygoma.

Heavy-impact forces or high-velocity injuries result in more extensive damage, leading to defects involving two or more orbital walls and extending into the posterior third of the orbit.

Treatment is directed at the precise anatomic reconstruction of the orbital shape and volume in order to restore the correct position of the eye.

We have observed three types of orbital-wall injuries, each requiring different reconstructive techniques:
- linear fractures,
- defects limited to one wall, usually the floor (the typical blow-out fracture),
- complex orbital-wall defects.

Linear Fractures

The thin bones of the medial and inferior orbital walls break like an eggshell, often leaving the fragments attached one to each other. A dent or a tub forms, causing enlargement of the orbit. In most cases, there is enough residual stability to allow filling with bone chips (see Case 7.1).

Dents and tubs are often observed in untreated orbital fractures (Chapter 8).

Blow-Out Fractures

In the literature, orbital floor blow-out fractures are the most extensively discussed type of orbital-wall injury. They are subdivided into pure (isolated) and impure blow-out fractures (associated with injuries to the orbital frame) [32]. Controversial theories about the pathologic mechanism leading to the defect have included hydraulic pressure [30] and buckling forces transmitted from the infraorbital rim to the orbital floor [78].

The indications for operative treatment have been discussed in Chapter 5.

Blow-out fractures are typically located in the anterior or middle part of the orbital floor, the defect being less than 2 cm in diameter. These defects may be bridged with a single onlay graft morticed over their edges. When the graft overlaps the defect by at least 5 mm, this usually obviates fixation.

The literature is replete with recommendations on materials to bridge these defects [91, 148–156]. Currently, we prefer resorbable polydioxanone sheets (PDS Ethicon), which are available in 0.25 mm and 0.5 mm thickness. PDS is well tolerated and to a large extent replaced by bone [91]. Alternatively, porous polyethylene (MEDPOR) [157] or shaved calvarial bone grafts with intact periosteum [158] may be used. Silastic sheets and lyophilized dura are materials that should no longer be used for the repair of orbital-wall fractures: The former has a high number of reported complications [159–163], and the latter lacks the mechanical stability necessary for bridging such defects.

Surgical exposure of the orbital floor is achieved through a lower eyelid incision. The defect is exposed, and the entrapped soft tissues are carefully elevated from the maxillary sinus. The edges of the defect are exposed until a circular bony platform has been established. Grafting of the defect follows stabilization of the associated orbital frame fractures, because reduction of the zygoma can alter the size of the orbital-floor defect. The graft is placed so as to overly the edges of the defect, and forced duction testing (Figure 4.10) is performed before and after grafting to confirm free mobility of the globe.

Complex Orbital-Wall Defects

A complex orbital-wall defect is characterized by its extension into the posterior third of the orbit and/or by involving two or more orbital walls. These defects are complicated by the following factors:
- The posterior bony ledge is very small and therefore does not offer support for grafts.
- Disruption of the periorbit with fat protruding on both sides of the retractors makes exposure and visibility difficult.

Early meticulous repair of these defects is of critical importance because inadequate reconstruction results in serious cosmetic and functional defects (see Chapter 8), which are difficult or impossible to correct completely. The initial treatment therefore must aim at total anatomic reconstruction of the bony orbit. A critical area for reconstruction is the postero-medial orbital wall (key area, see Chapter 2), which is essential for supporting the globe in its antero-posterior position. Inadequate reconstruction of this area leads to enophthalmos and eventually diplopia. It is our clinical impression that this site requires a greater mechanical stability than other areas of the orbital wall. A 2 x 2 cm defect of the orbital roof, for example, may still be bridged with a PDS sheet, whereas in this key area the sheet would bulge into the maxillary sinus, leading to increased orbital volume.

Basic Considerations

Although every complex orbital fracture presents with its own difficulties, basic principles allow for a systematic approach, thereby saving operating time and optimizing the final result. We consider the following points to be important:
- *Exposure:* Radical exposure of all defects is the basis of anatomic reconstruction. Complex fractures usually require a 360° subperiosteal dissection of the orbit back into the posterior cone. The importance of adequate exposure cannot be over-emphasized.
- *Segmental reconstruction:* Large defects extending over two or more walls are reconstructed with several individual grafts. With the techniques presently available, it would be virtually impossible to reproduce the complex three-dimensional shape of a large defect with a single graft, not to mention the difficulties involved in inserting such a graft into the orbit without damaging the eye and adnexae.
- *Rigid fixation:* Defects in the postero-medial wall (key area) are particularly difficult to deal with, because there is little or no support for bone grafts available. Based on the principle of rigid fixation for the internal orbit [16], a specially designed plate (Figure 7.17) or a cantilevered bone graft (Figure 7.18) can be used to construct a stable posterior platform, which converts a large defect into two smaller ones and at the same time serves as a scaffold for bone grafting of the remaining defects. These grafts can usually be wedged in without further fixation.
- *Enhancement of visibility:* Visibility and access to the deep orbit is difficult because of the narrow space and is further impaired by orbital fat protruding on both sides of the retractors (Figure 7.18). It can be enhanced by inserting a flexible sheet into the orbit after completion of the subperiosteal dissection [164] (Figures 7.18 and 7.19). The sheet replaces the periorbit and prevents extrusion of fat. We use a resorbable sheet for this purpose (polydioxanone, PDS Ethicon), which is left in situ as a bridging material for small defects between the bone grafts.
- *Sequence:* From the points mentioned above it is evident that reconstruction of a complex wall defect is initiated with the insertion of a graft for reconstructing the postero-medial wall.
- *Overcorrection:* During the first 4 to 6 months after orbital reconstruction, the globe sinks back to a certain degree. The pathomechanisms responsible include dissolution of edema, bone-graft resorption [165], and possibly fat atrophy. The change in eye position occurs predominantly in the antero-posterior direction, whereas the vertical position remains essentially unchanged. Therefore, overcorrection in the antero-posterior axis (not in the vertical) should be achieved during surgery. According to our clinical impression, 2–3 mm of overcorrection is adequate, although objective data are not yet available [166].

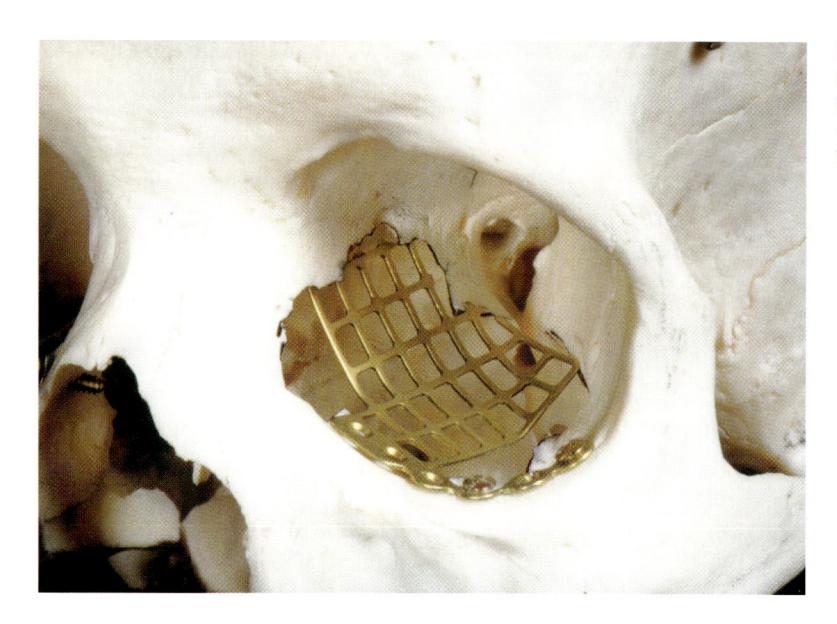

Figure 7.16. Rigid fixation of the internal orbit with an orbital plate. The plate is fixed to the anterior orbital rim and provides a stable platform for additional bone-graft reconstruction of the orbit.

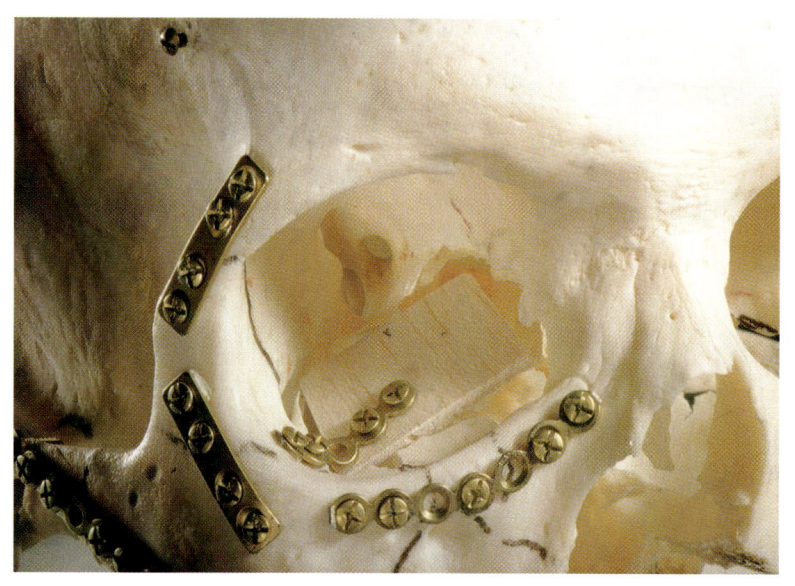

Figure 7.17. Rigid fixation of the internal orbit with a cantilevered calvarial bone graft. A 2 x 3 cm piece of calvarial bone is cantilevered to the infraorbital rim with a miniplate. The graft does not overlap the edges of the defect, and it is oriented in such a manner as to reconstruct the posteromedial wall. It serves as a strut to give support to additional bone grafts.

Figure 7.18 (a, b). (a) The ruptured periorbit protrudes on both sides of the malleable retractor, making access and visibility difficult. (b) A resorbable sheet (PDS Ethicon) improves visibility during surgery and is adequate to bridge small defects. It prevents herniation of orbital fat around the malleable retractor and avoids impingment of the graft into the periorbit (see also Figure 7.19).

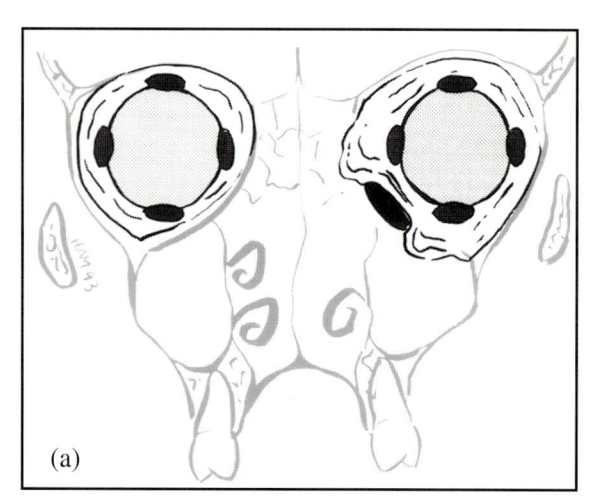

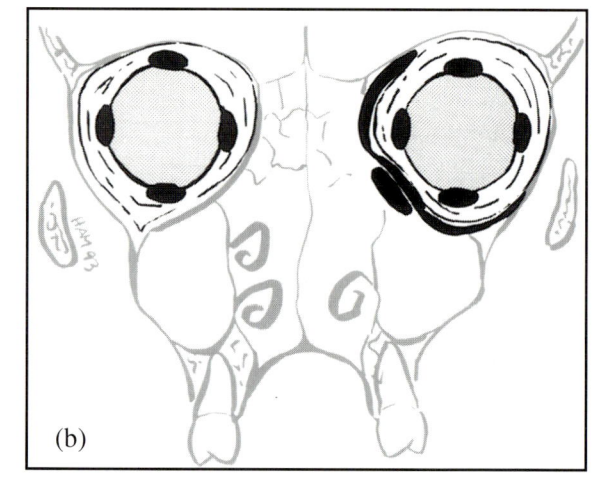

(a)

(b)

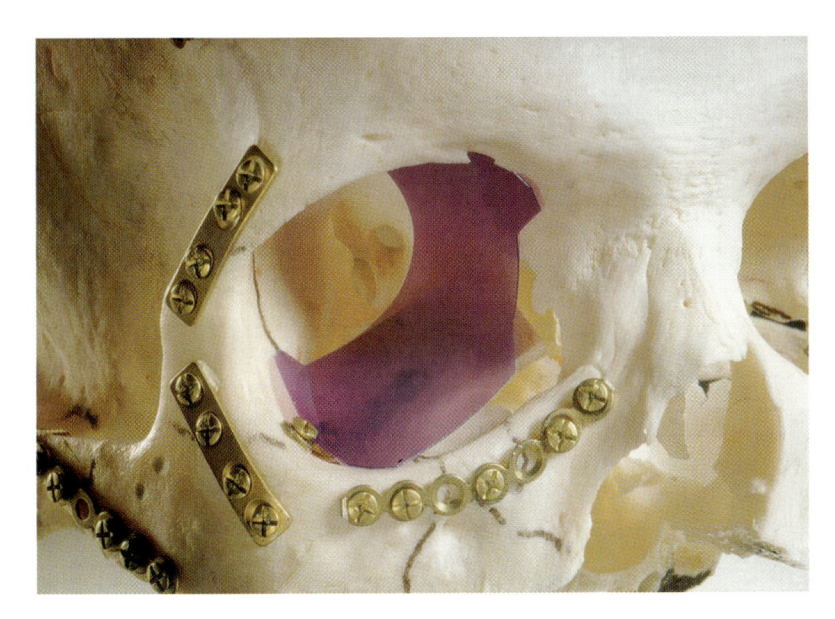

Figure 7.19. Reconstruction of a complex orbital fracture using a cantilevered bone graft and a flexible, resorbable sheet (PDS Ethicon).

7.5 Surgical Technique for the Repair of Complex Orbital Fractures

Repair of complex orbital fractures involving all parts of the orbit requires a combination of all the techniques described above. The sequence is as follows:
- exposure of the entire area involved in the fracture;
- reconstruction of the orbital frame, initiated with the positioning of the zygoma (outer orbital frame) and followed by reconstruction of the inner orbital frame;
- with an intact orbital frame, reconstruction of the orbital wall defects according to the principles outlined in Section 7.4.

For exposure, both coronal and lower eyelid incisions are used in most cases, combined with an intraoral approach. After developing the coronal flap and exposing the zygomatic arch, one begins subperiosteal dissection of the orbit at an uninjured site of the orbit, usually the upper lateral wall. Along the lateral wall, dissection is carried down to the inferior orbital fissure, exposing the articulation between the zygoma and the greater wing of the sphenoid (landmark 1 in Figure 7.10), which is essential for correct positioning of the zygomatic body. The next step is to completely detach the periorbit of the displaced zygoma, including the lateral canthal ligament.

Upon dissection of the orbital floor, several small arteries arising from the infraorbital neurovascular bundle to the periorbit often need to be coagulated.

After completion of the exposure of the orbital floor and the lateral orbital wall, the connective tissue of the inferior orbital fissure, which prevents a clear identification of the transition between floor and lateral wall, is divided after thorough bipolar coagulation.

Dissection of the medial orbital wall starts again at the orbital roof and proceeds inferiorly. The anterior ethmoid artery is transsected. Starting from the coronal approach, the posterior bony ledge of the deep orbital cone is exposed. If any difficulty arises in exposing the deep orbit in this area, a superior marginotomy (Figure 7.7) is advisable.

The exposure is sufficient when the triangular groove formed by the posterior medial bony ledge and the intact posterior part of the lateral wall (see Figure 2.1) becomes visible. Upon completion of the dissection, the flexible PDS sheet replacing the periorbit is inserted along the medial wall from the coronal to the infraorbital incision.

Three-dimensional reconstruction of the orbital frame is now performed, beginning with positioning of the zygoma as described in Section 7.2, followed by stabilization of the inner orbital frame. Then, orbital-wall reconstruction is started with reconstruction of the posteromedial wall according to the principles outlined in Section 7.4. Correct positioning of the orbital plate or cantilevered bone graft is of vital importance. It should be kept in mind that this graft is angulated in two planes, ascending from anterior to posterior (Figure 7.17). The graft reconstructing the key area is usually easier to insert if it does not overlap the defect, but rather is aligned just flush with its lateral edges. This can be done inasmuch as mechanical support by the posterior bone ledge is unnecessary.

Additional bone grafts are inserted where appropriate. For example, the superior portion of the medial wall and the inferior orbital fissure often need additional support. Small residual defects are adequately reconstructed with the PDS sheet. Upon completion of the reconstruction, the globe should exhibit an approximately 2-mm overcorrection in the antero-posterior direction, whereas the vertical position should be set as desired. Finally, a forced duction test is performed to ascertain free mobility of the globe.

If a direct canthopexy has been prepared, it is now tightened, and then the lateral canthal ligament is reattached to the medial aspect of the lateral orbital rim, which is best achieved with a transosseous suture. The reconstruction is completed with resuspension of the soft tissues and closure of the incisions.

Basic Steps in Complex Orbital-Fracture Repair
– Generous exposure of the entire area involved in the trauma
– Insertion of a flexible sheet
– Reconstruction of the orbital frame
– Reconstruction of the key area using rigid fixation
– Additional grafts for the remaining defects
– (Medial canthopexy if necessary)
– Lateral canthopexy, soft tissue resuspension

7.6 Case Reports

Case 7.1 (Figure 7.20 a–h)
Fragmented Orbito-Zygomatic Fracture

A 29-year-old female patient riding a bycicle was hit by a car, leading to a left orbitozygomatic fracture with associated Le Fort I fracture (a, b, c). Three-dimensional reconstruction of the orbital frame was performed (d, e, f), using a combination of coronal, mid-eyelid and intraoral approach. A dent in the posterior floor was grafted with calvarial bone chips (d, f).

One year after one-stage reconstruction (g, h), the patient had normal binocular vision.

Exposure of the sphenozygomatic fracture line (i) is necessary to assess the correct reduction of the zygomatic body.

Figure 7.20 (a-c). Case 7.1: Schematic drawing (a) and CT scans (b, c) of a left orbito-zygomatic fracture Type IV.

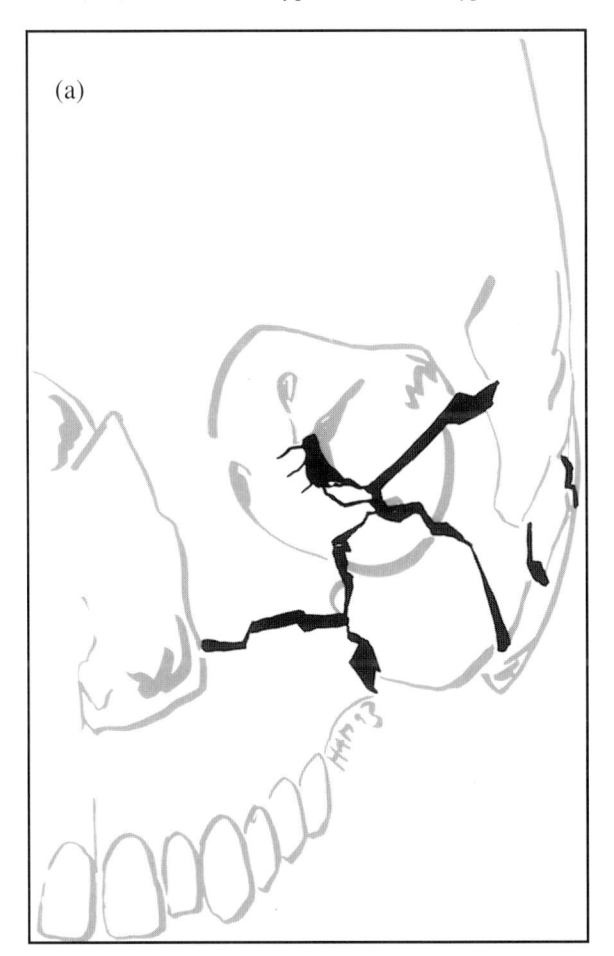

Comments
– Plating of the fracture line at the lateral orbital wall (c, i) may be helpful in cases of fragmentation of the zygomatic body. It perfectly stabilizes the lateral orbital rim fragment, thereby providing a reliable platform for reduction of the zygomatic body and the maxilla.
– Dents in the posterior part of the orbital floor are frequent and may lead to widening of the infraorbital fissure and enophthalmos. Filling with bone chips is sufficient if there is no real defect.

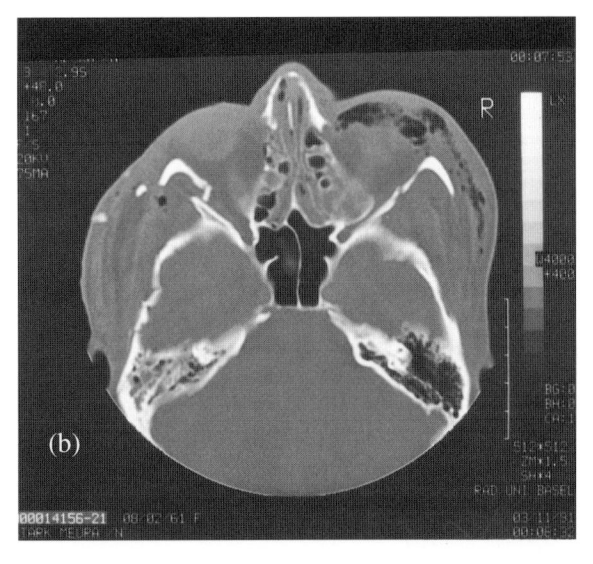

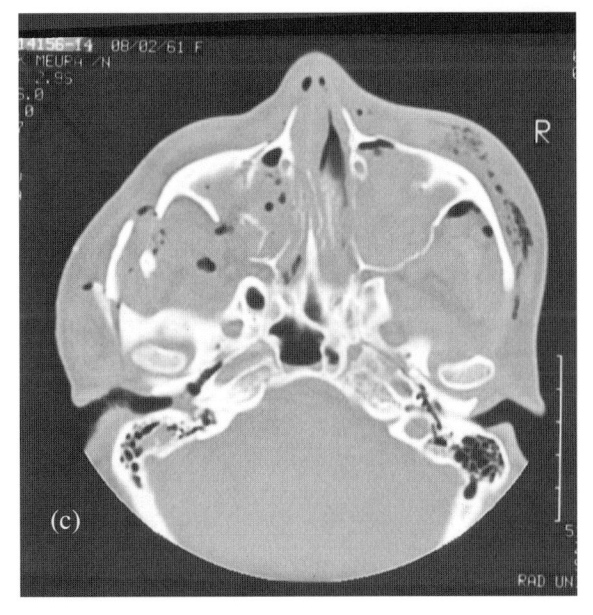

Figure 7.20 (d-f). Case 7.1: Repair of an orbito-zygomatic fracture Type IV. Schematic drawing (d) and CT scans (e, f).

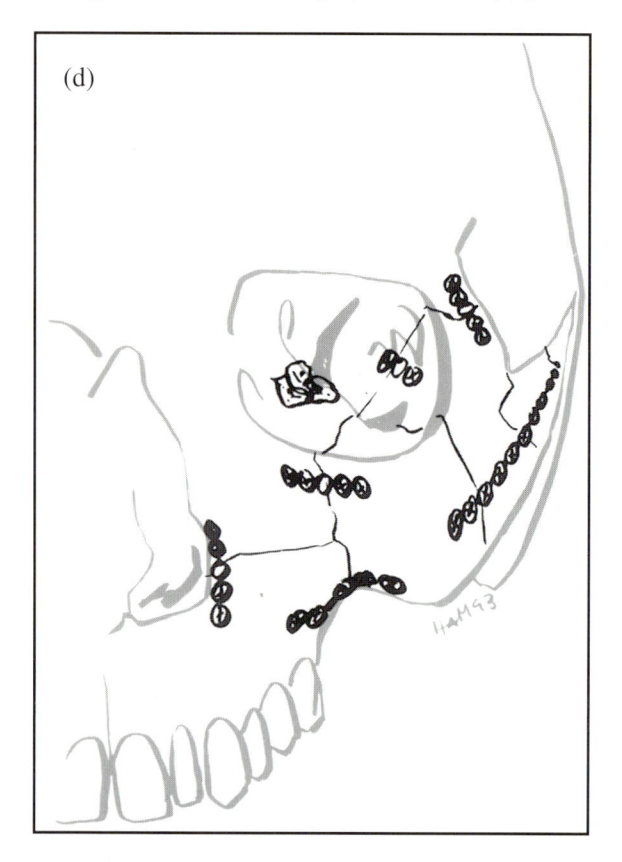

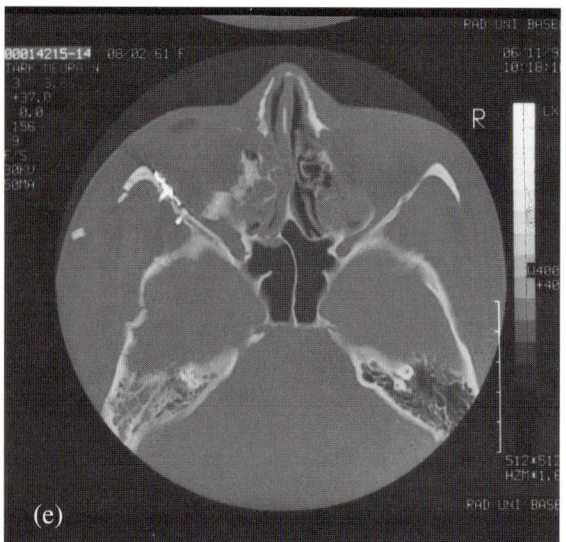

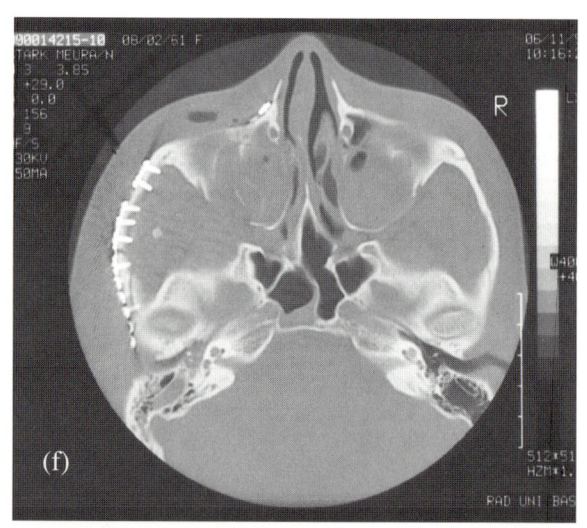

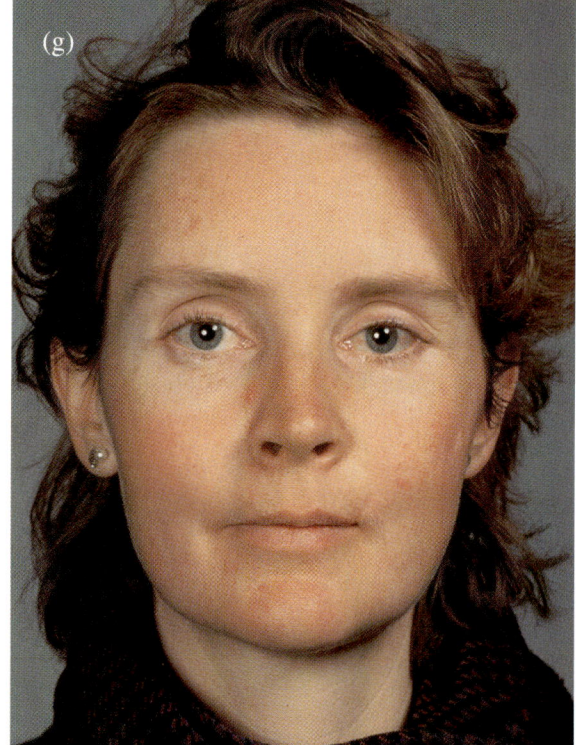

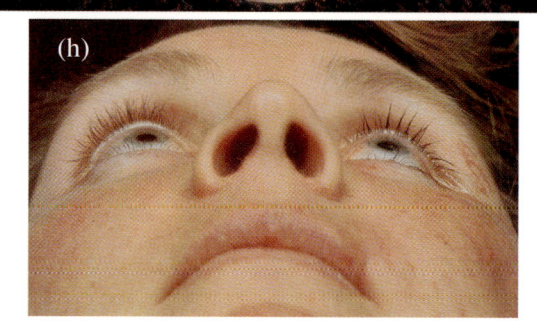

Figure 7.20 (g, h). Case 7.1: The patient 1 year after orbital reconstruction using craniofacial techniques.

Figure 7.20 (i). Case 7.1: Exposure and plating of the lateral orbital wall (spheno-zygomatic suture).

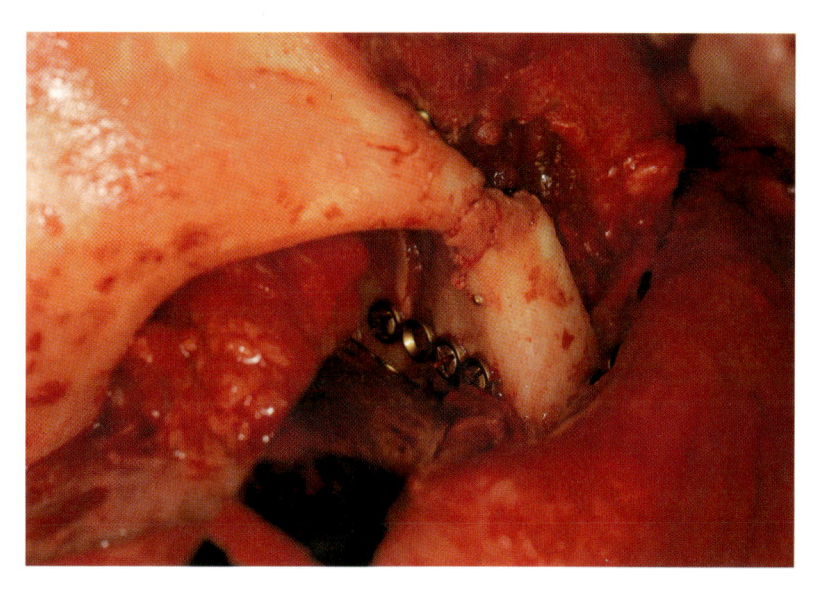

Case 7.2 (Figure 7.21 a–h)
Complex Orbital Fracture with Two-Wall Defect

A 20-year-old female patient was hit by a car, leading to a complex left orbital fracture involving the outer frame and the internal orbit. In addition to displacement of the zygoma, there was a defect in the floor and medial wall extending deep into the posterior cone and thus involving the key area (a, b, c). Repair was performed through a combination of coronal, mid-lower eyelid, and intraoral incisions. After three-dimensional reconstruction of the outer orbital frame, the postero-medial wall defect was reconstructed with a cantilevered calvarial bone graft (d). A flexible PDS sheet was used to enhance visibility and to bridge small remaining defects in the upper medial wall and the infraorbital fissure. The arrow in (e) shows the sheet.

The calvarial graft reproduced the ascending plane of the postero-medial wall (f).

Nine months after one-stage reconstruction (g, h), the patient had normal binocular vision except for extreme upward gaze.

Comment
There is minimal orbital enlargement in the upper medial part (e). In this area (arrow in d) an additional bone graft would have been helpful.

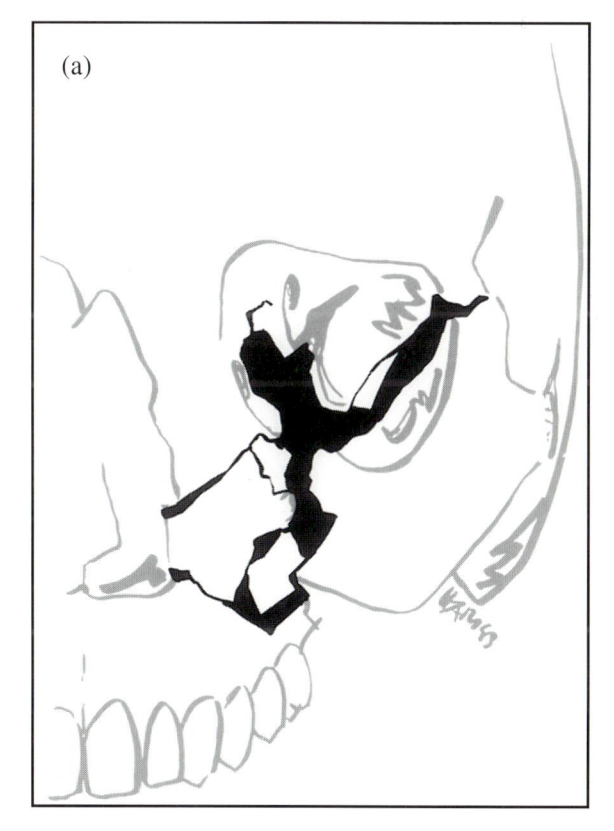

Figure 7.21 (a-c). Case 7.2: Schematic drawing (a) and CT scans (b, c) of a left orbito-zygomatic fracture Type IV with a two-wall defect involving the key area.

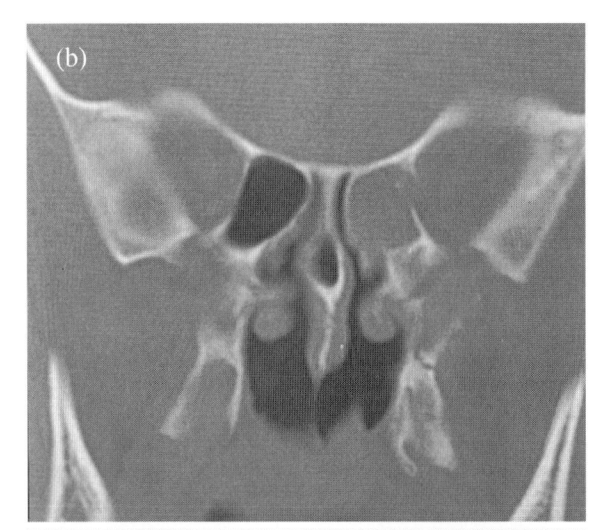

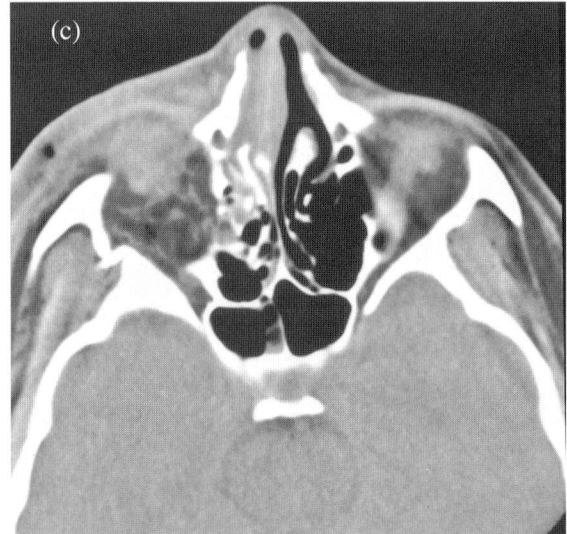

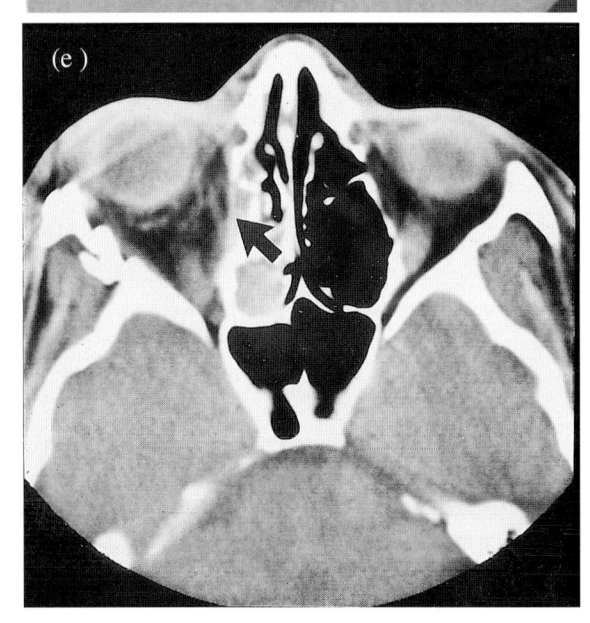

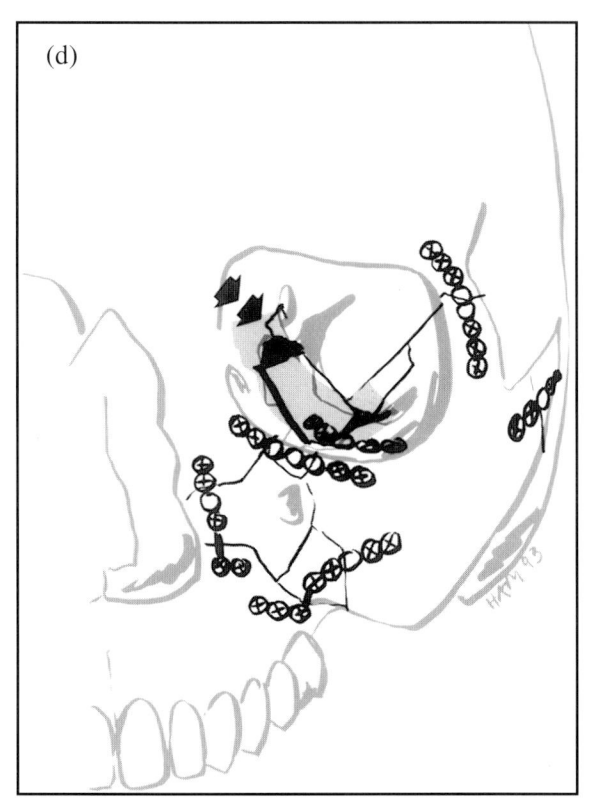

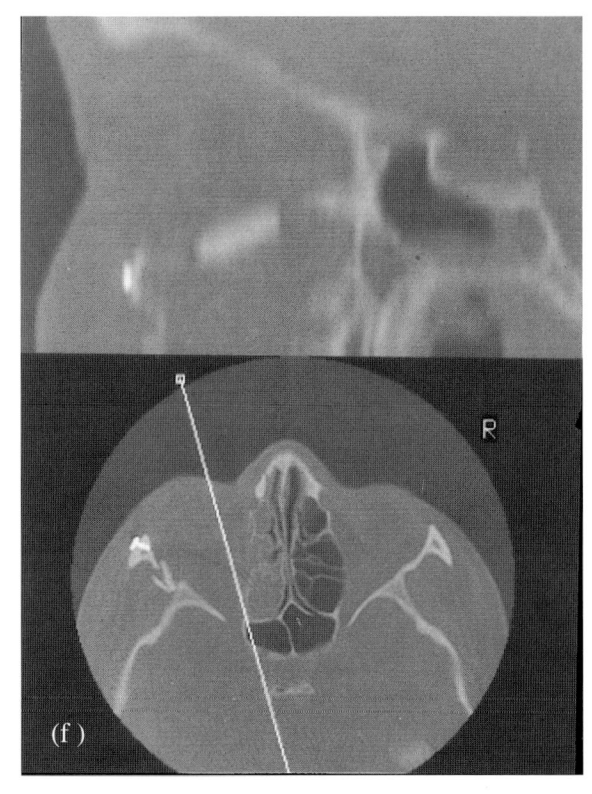

Figure 7.21 (d-f). Case 7.2: Fracture repair using a cantilevered bone graft for rigid fixation of the internal orbit. Schematic drawing (d) and CT scans (e, f).

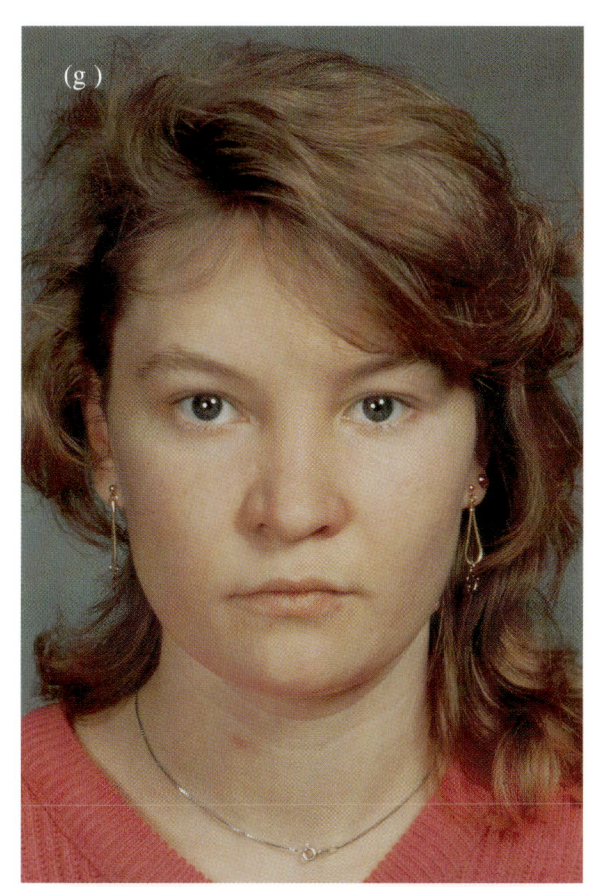

Figure 7.21 (g, h). Case 7.2: The patient 9 months after orbital reconstruction using craniofacial techniques and rigid fixation for the internal orbit.

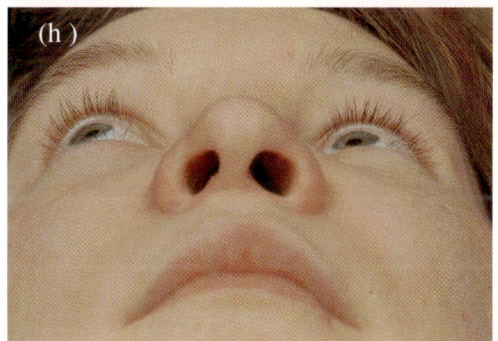

Case 7.3 (Figure 7.22 a–f)
Naso-Orbito-Ethmoid Injury Type III

This 47-year-old patient was involved in a car accident. Upon admission, a naso-orbito-ethmoid fracture Type III with cerebrospinal fluid rhinorrhea was diagnosed (a). The intercanthal distance was 43 mm.

He was operated on on the 4th day after admission. The fractures were exposed through a combination of coronal and lower eyelid approaches. Bilateral superior marginotomies were performed to permit inspection of the anterior cranial base, where a dural leak on the right side was repaired. There was no sizable central fragment, so bilateral direct canthopexy was performed after reconstruction of the inner orbital frame (b, c). Nasal reconstruction was done with an outer table graft, the tip of the graft being inserted between the alar cartilages.

The patient is shown before (d) and 7 months after one-stage reconstruction (e); intercanthal distance is 36 mm.

Comment
Use of a miniplate as an insertion point allows precise placement of the transnasal canthopexy, which must be placed posterior to the lacrimal crest (f).

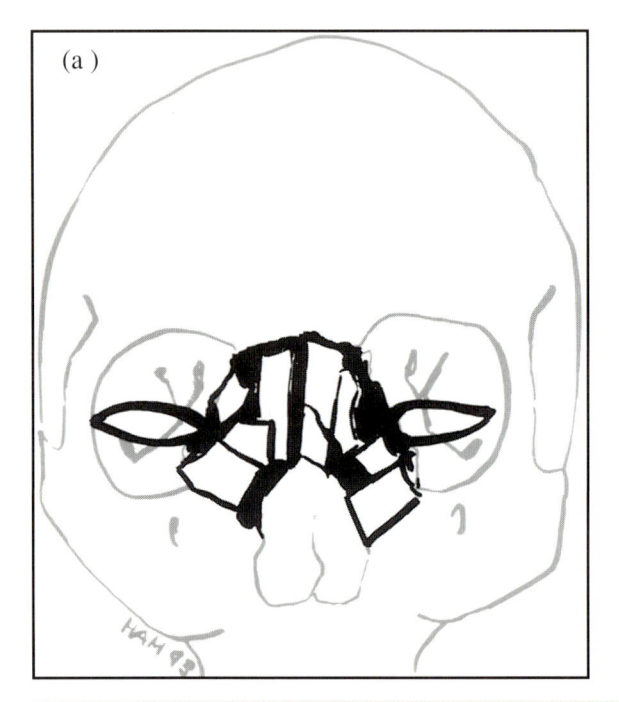

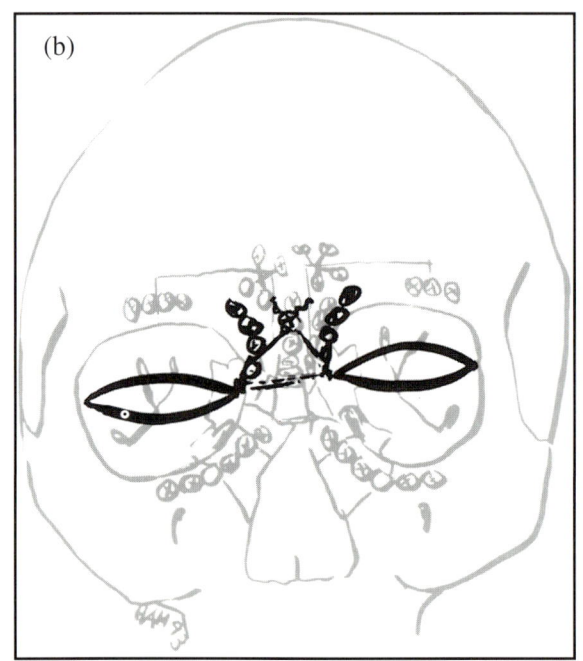

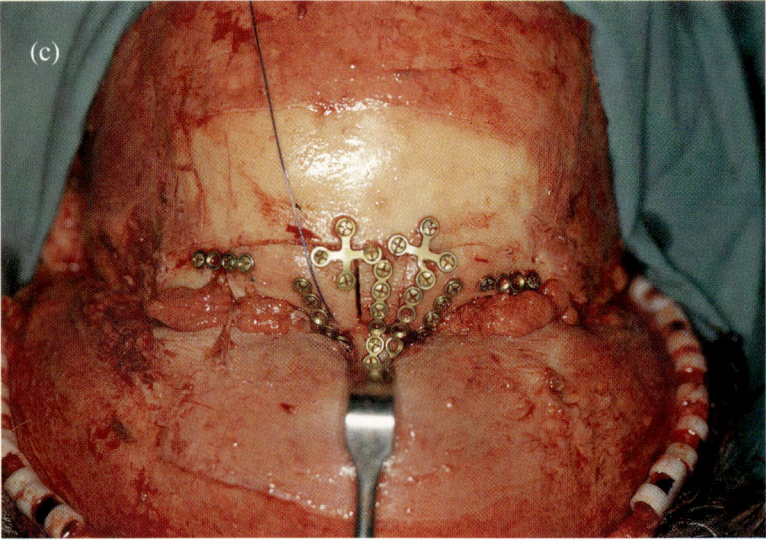

Figure 7.22 (a, b). Case 7.3: Schematic drawings of a naso-orbito-ethmoid fracture Type III (a) and of repair (b).

Figure 7.22 (c). Case 7.3: Repair of a naso-orbito-ethmoid fracture Type III, intraoperative view.

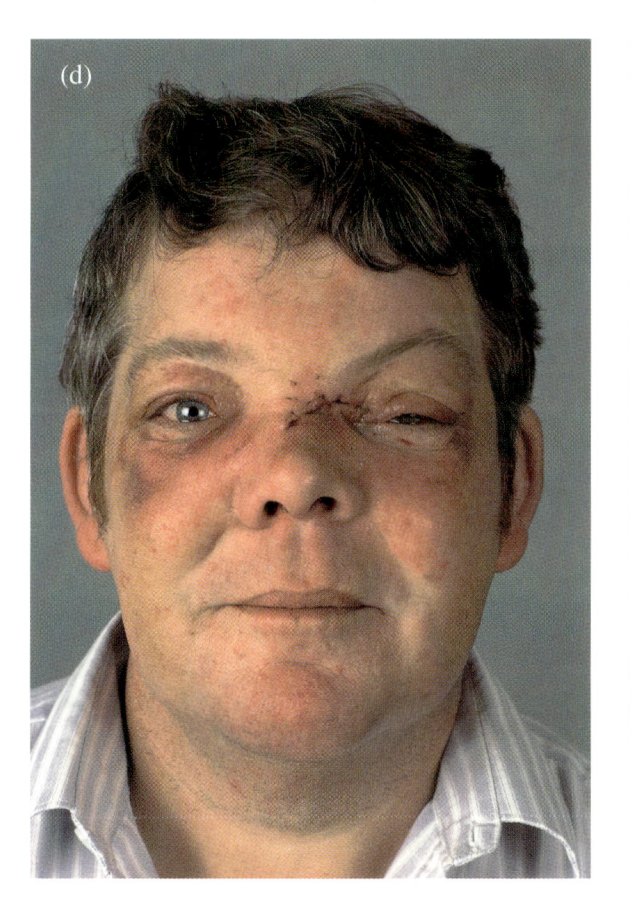

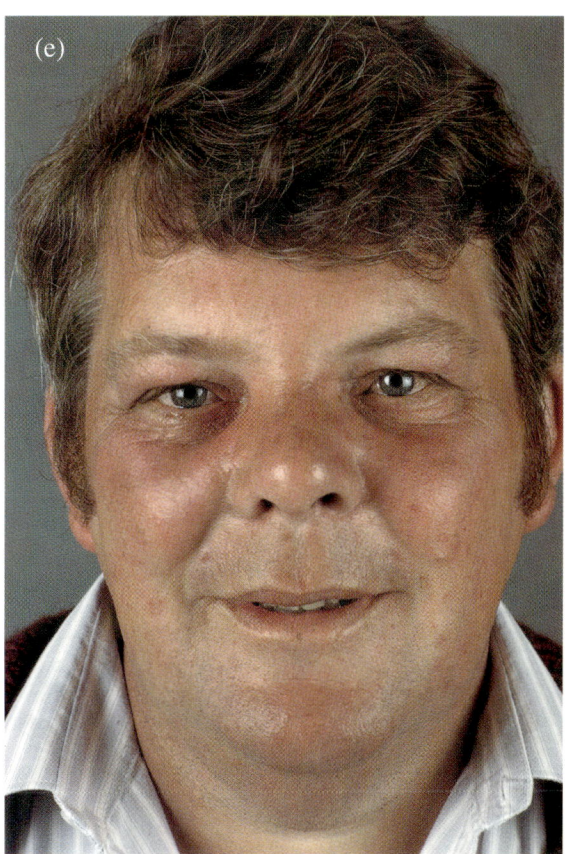

Figure 7.22 (d, e). Case 7.3: The patient before (d) and 7 months after one-stage reconstruction (e).

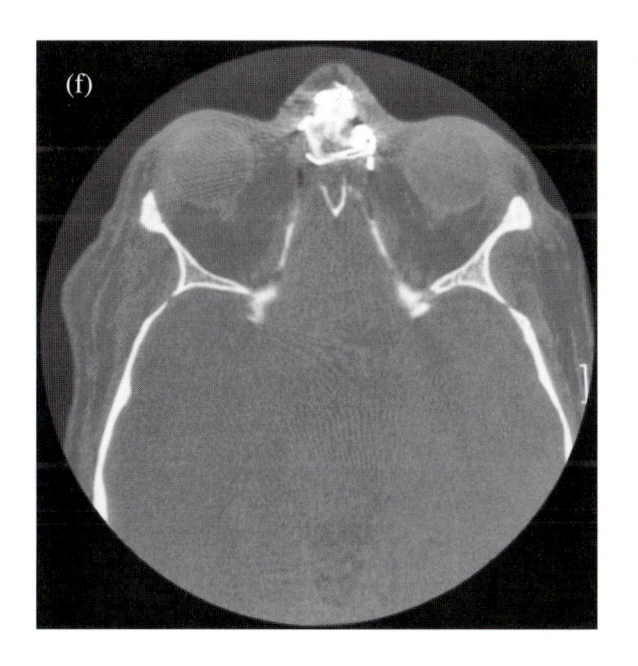

Figure 7.22 (f). Case 7.3: Use of a miniplate to create the insertion point of the transnasal canthopexy.

Case 7.4 (Figure 7.23 a–f)
Complex Naso-Orbito-Ethmoid Fracture with Avulsion of the Left Globe

This 50-year-old patient was hit by a falling tractor resulting in a severe open midface and naso-orbito-ethmoid fracture with avulsion of the left globe and loss of the entire nasal skeleton (a, b). The outer facial frame, however, remained intact.

Following tracheostomy, the midfacial buttress system was reconstructed, starting concentrically from the intact zygomas. The nasal skeleton was reconstructed with calvarial bone grafts. Following enucleation of the avulsed globe, the orbital floor and medial wall were reconstructed with a flag-shaped orbital plate (c), as shown in Figure 7.17. Prior to insertion of the plate, the ethmoidal roof (anterior skull base) was inspected from below, revealing no defect.

The plate was generously packed with bone chips in order to compensate for the volume of the globe (d). A space holder was inserted into the conjunctival sac, which was temporarily closed with sutures for 2 weeks.

The patient is shown 11 months after one-stage orbital reconstruction and insertion of a left eye prosthesis (e). Two secondary procedures were performed for nasal obstruction.

Comment
In this patient, the entire lower half of the left orbit had to be replaced. In our view, there was virtually no reconstructive alternative to the titanium orbital plate in this case.

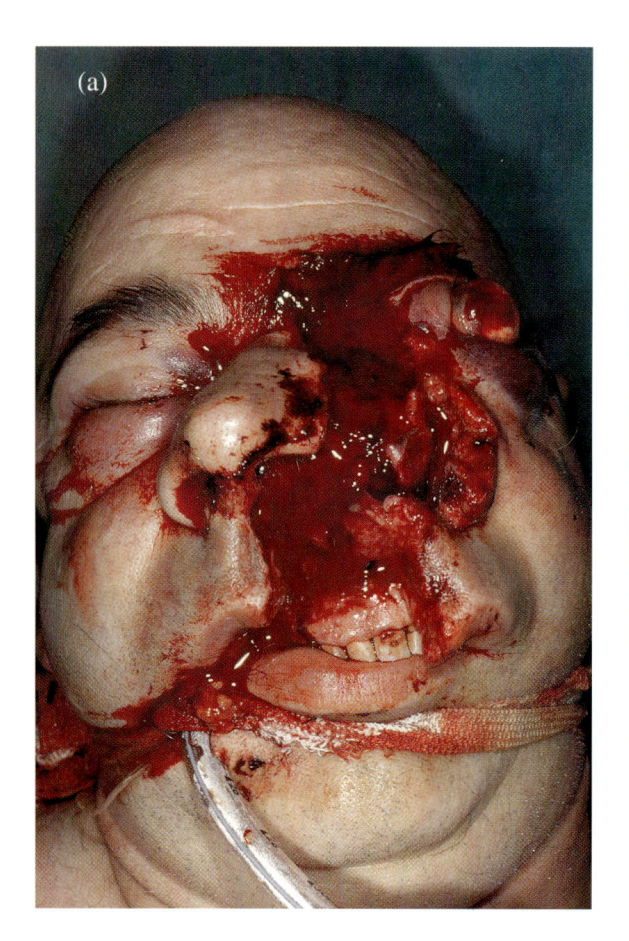

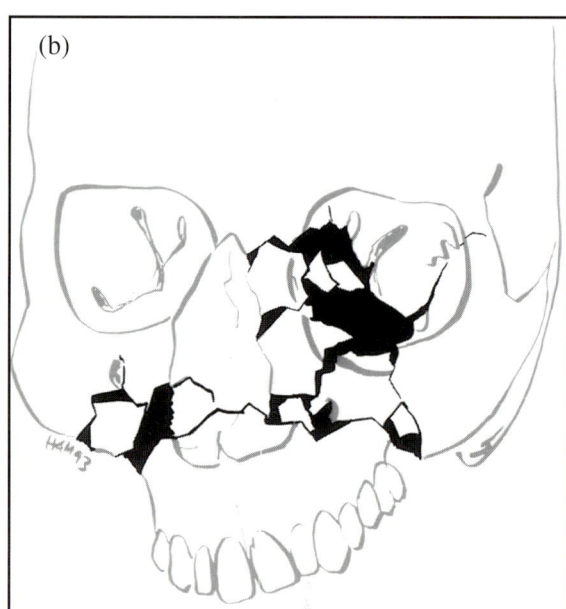

Figure 7.23 (a, b). Case 7.4: Combined left orbital fracture with avulsion of the ocular globe. Destruction of the entire left orbital floor and medial wall and the nasal skeleton.

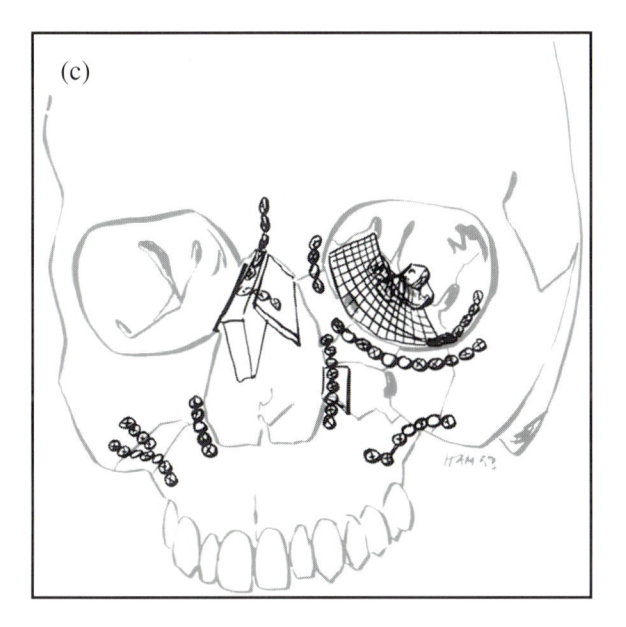

Figure 7.23 (c, d). Case 7.4: (c) Repair of the left orbit using a flag shaped orbital plate, packed with bone grafts. (d) The patient 11 months after one-stage reconstruction.

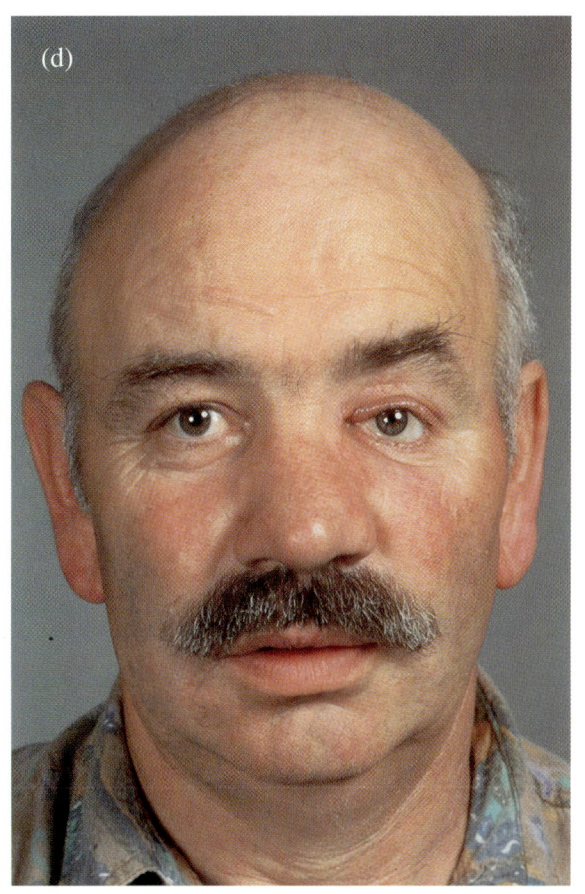

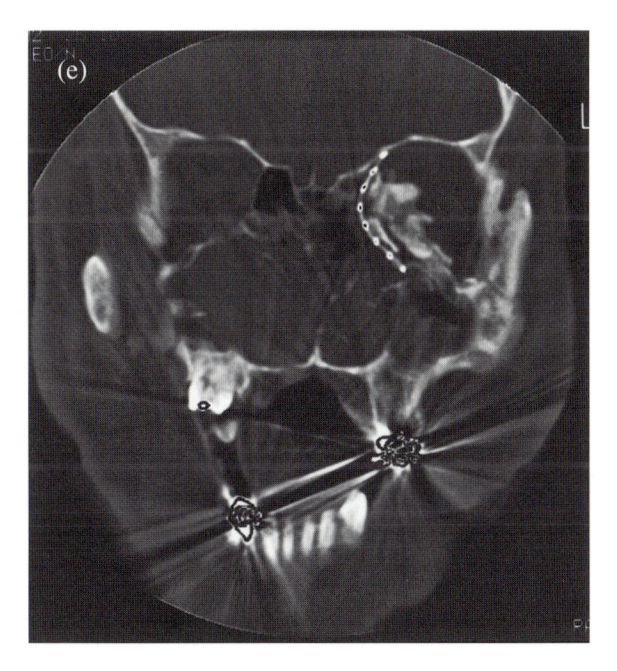

Figure 7.23 (e). Case 7.4: Extensive bone grafting to the orbit was performed in order to compensate for the volume of the avulsed globe.

Case 7.5 (Figure 7.24 a–m)
Complex Four-Wall Fracture of the Right Orbit with Cranial Base Injury and Dural Laceration

A 16-year-old patient (a) after a fall from a mountain bike onto his head, with open and sand-contaminated calvarial, orbital, and skull base fractures (b, c, d, e, f).

There was an nondisplaced fracture running through the left optic canal. The swinging flash light

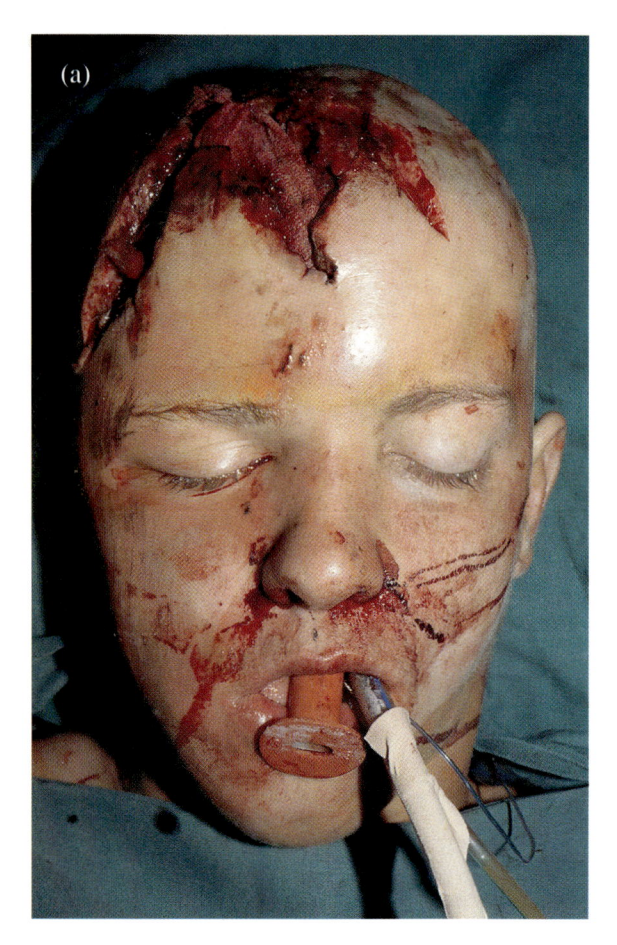

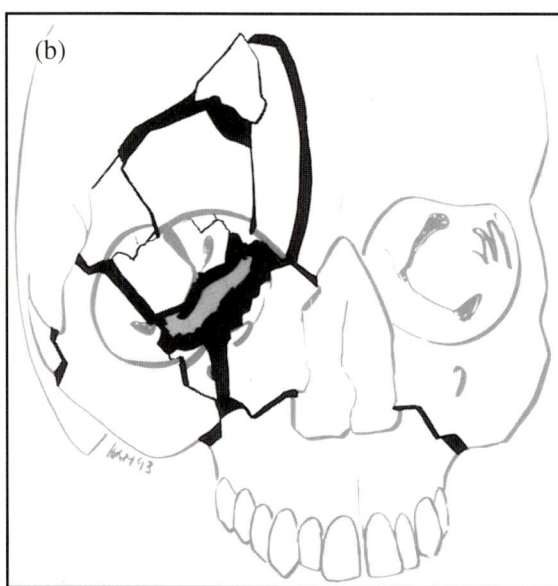

Figure 7.24 (a, b). Case 7.5: Complex fracture of the left orbit involving all four walls.

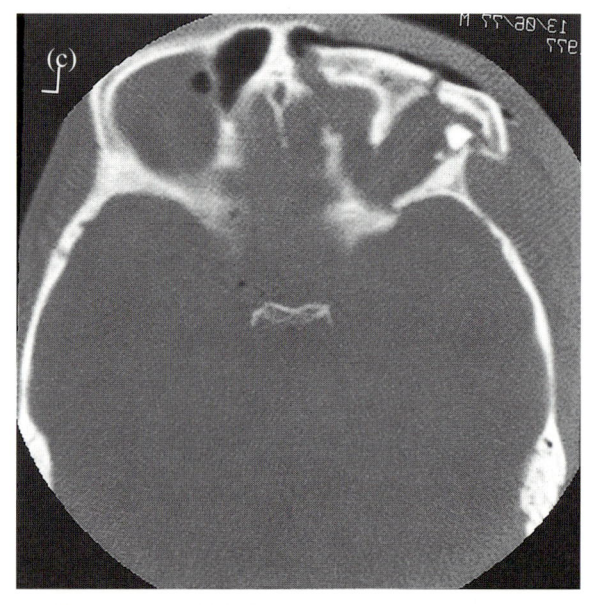

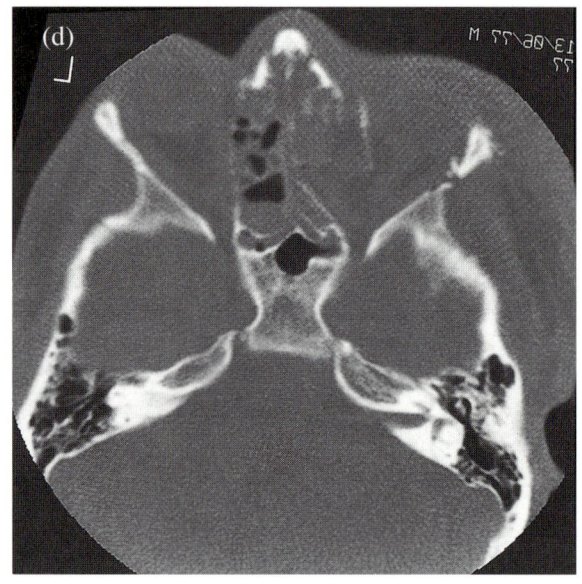

Figure 7.24 (c, d). Case 7.5: CT scans of the fracture involving the entire orbit.

test, however, was normal, so that no decompressive surgery was undertaken (see also Figure 4.7).

Exposure of the fracture was achieved through modified coronal, mid-lower eyelid, and intraoral incisions. After temporary removal of the calvarial and supraorbital bone fragments, revision of the anterior skull base with duraplasty was performed. Bony reconstruction was begun with positioning of the zygomatic body, the landmarks being the greater sphenoid wing and the zygomatic arch (g). Stabilization of the zygomatic body was done with a plate inside the orbit. A resorbable sheet (PDS Ethicon) was inserted to replace the ruptured periorbit and to obliterate remaining gaps between bone grafts.

The postero-medial wall was reconstructed with a cantilevered bone graft, and the calvarial and supraorbital rim fragments were replaced (h, i, j, k). Additional bone grafts were inserted as fillers.

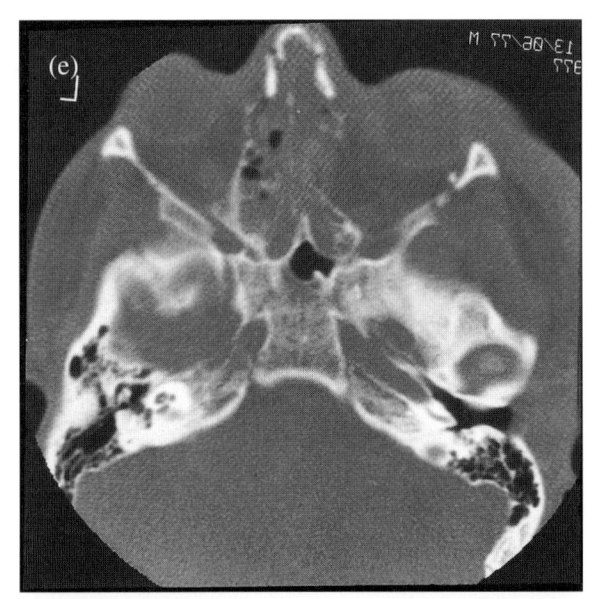

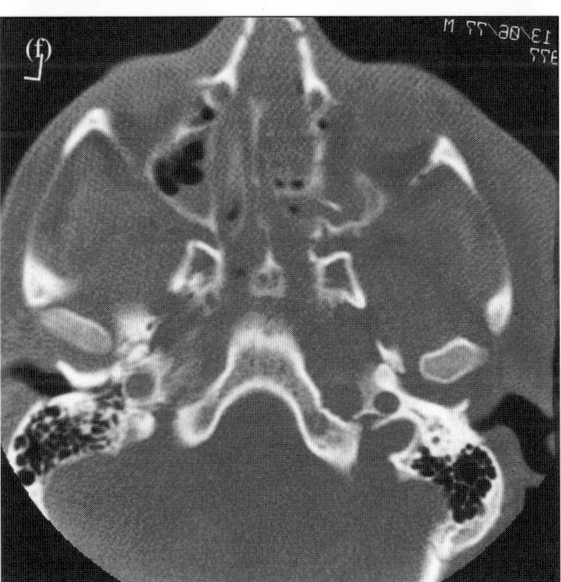

Figure 7.24 (e, f). Case 7.5: CT scans of the fracture involving the entire orbit.

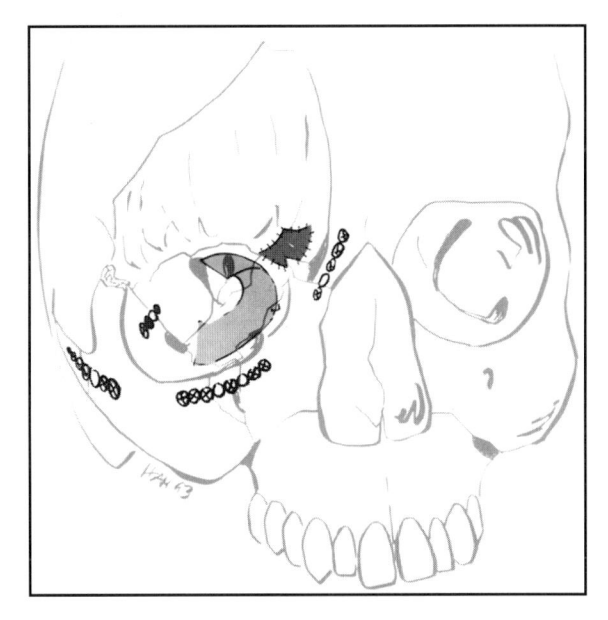

Figure 7.24 (g). Case 7.5: First stage of fracture repair. Positioning of the zygoma using the lateral orbital wall and the zygomatic arch as landmarks. The ruptured periorbit is replaced with a flexible sheet. The dural leak has been repaired with a patch.

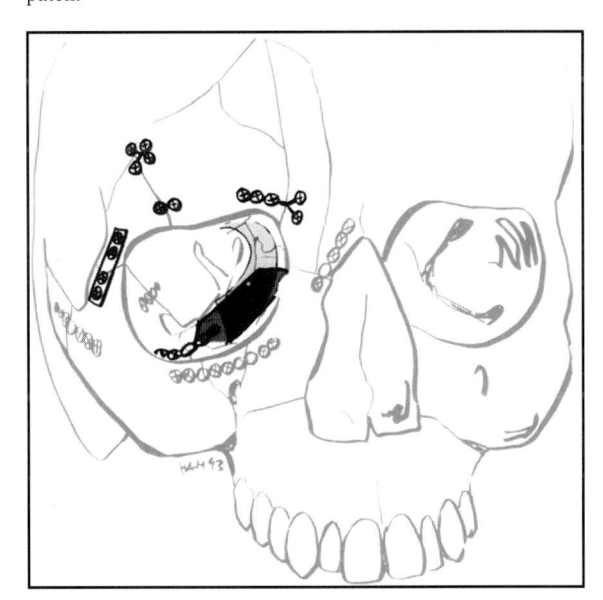

Figure 7.24 (h). Case 7.5: Completed fracture repair. The key area has been reconstructed with a cantilevered bone graft.

The patient 5 months after one-stage reconstruction (l, m): There is a 2-mm vertical malposition of the right globe and a 2-mm enophthalmos. Both eyes have full visual acuity, and there is no diplopia.

Comment
Retrospectively, reconstruction of the postero-medial wall would have been done preferably with an orbital plate instead of a cantilevered bone graft. This is because the orbital plate permits some bending.

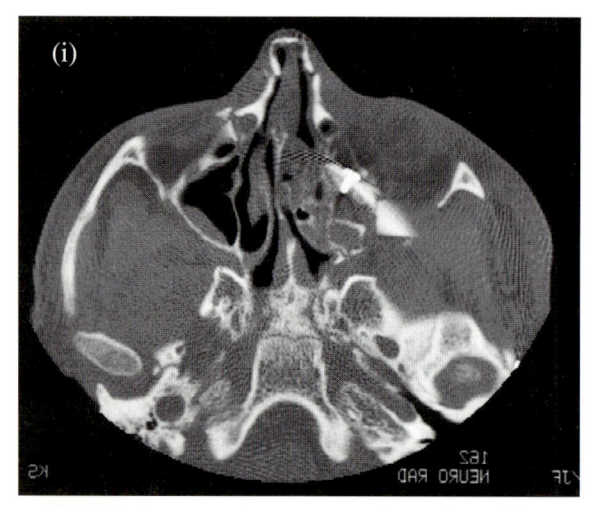

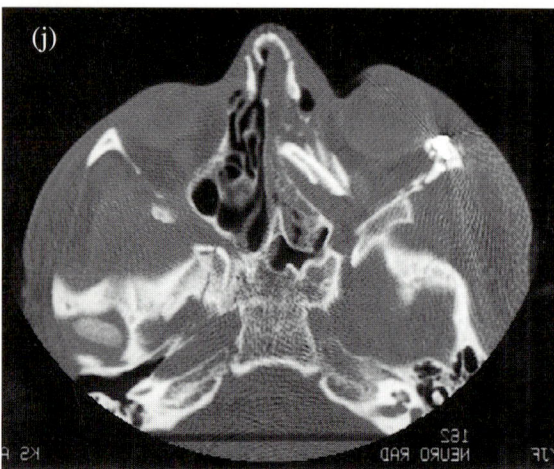

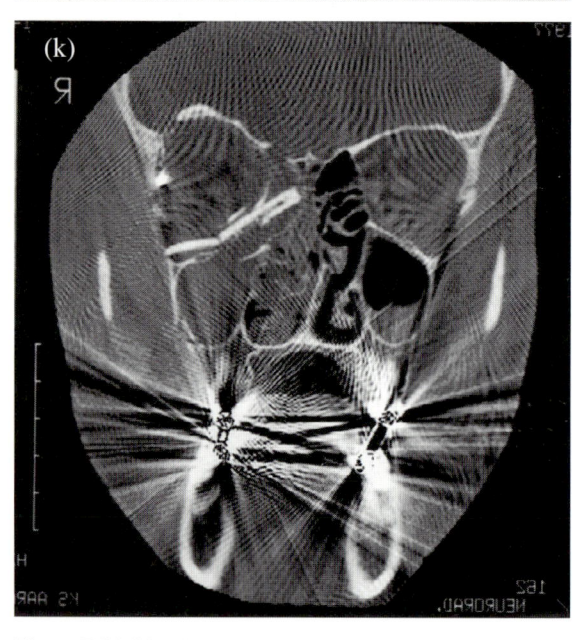

Figure 7.24 (i-k). Case 7.5: The cantilevered bone graft reconstructing the key area.

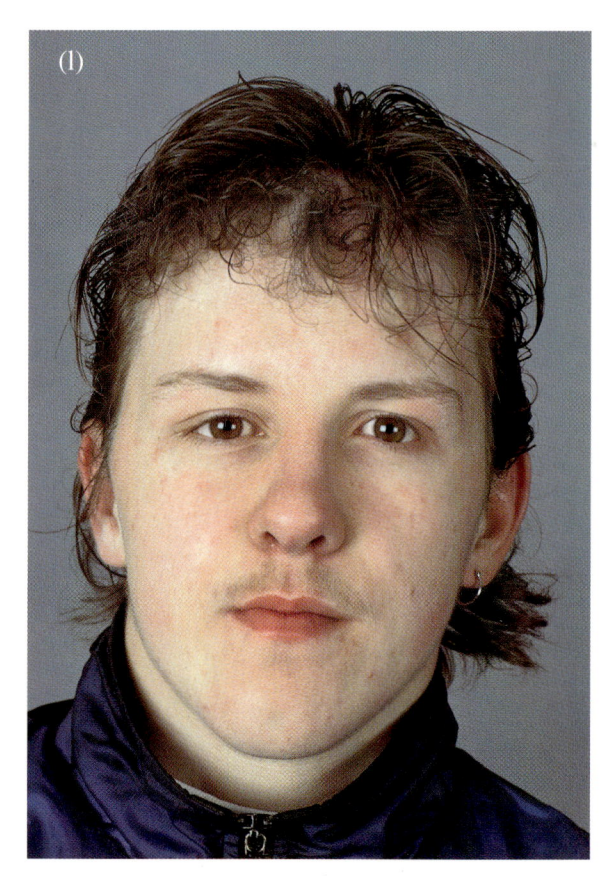

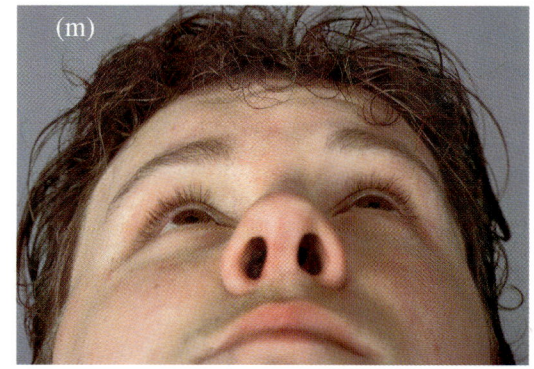

Figure 7.24 (l, m). Case 7.5: The patient 5 months after one-stage orbital reconstruction There is a 2-mm enophthalmos and 2-mm vertical malposition of the globe, but no diplopia.

7.7 Errors in Orbital Reconstruction

Reconstruction of the severely injured orbit is technically difficult, with possible sources of error occurring along the entire pathway of management. In order to avoid unfavorable results, a few basic points need to be emphasized.

Exposure

- Inadequate exposure is a common error in orbital reconstruction, often due to inadequate diagnosis of the severity of the injury. It is important to note that even large orbital-wall defects may initially reveal few clinical symptoms. CT evaluation is the method of choice to obtain reliable information about orbital injuries.
- The indication for an extended approach should be strongly considered. According to our experience, about 30% of all fractures involving the orbit benefit from a coronal approach.
- Before placing any plate or graft, the entire fracture pattern must be visually identified and the edges of any orbital wall defect must be completely exposed.

Orbital Frame

- Inadequate three-dimensional reduction of the orbital frame again is mostly due to inadequate exposure. For reduction of the zygomatic body, the alignment with the greater sphenoid wing is the most important landmark (Figure 7.10). Malpositioning the zygoma is always associated with a gap in the lateral orbital wall (see Figure 8.1).
- Fractures of the inner orbital frame usually require an extended (coronal) approach in order to ensure the correct rotational position of the central fragment (see Section 7.3).

Orbital Wall Reconstruction

Because of limited access and visibility, bridging of complex orbital wall defects is a highly difficult task. Some important errors in bone grafting are described below:

- No graft should be placed without adequate posterior support. Rigid fixation must be used, especially if no reliable posterior bony ledge can be identified (Figure 7.25).
- It is very difficult if not impossible to bridge a large defect with a single graft. With increasing size of the graft, its shaping and insertion become progressively more difficult (Figures 7.26 and 7.27). The rigid fixation techniques for the internal orbit described in Section 7.4 allow for the utilization of smaller grafts, which are easier to shape and to insert.
- Because of the complex shape of the orbit, a rigid graft laid onto the edges of a defect cannot be adequately fitted and therefore protrudes into the orbit (Figure 7.28). The graft must be wedged between the edges of the defect, possibly using rigid fixation.

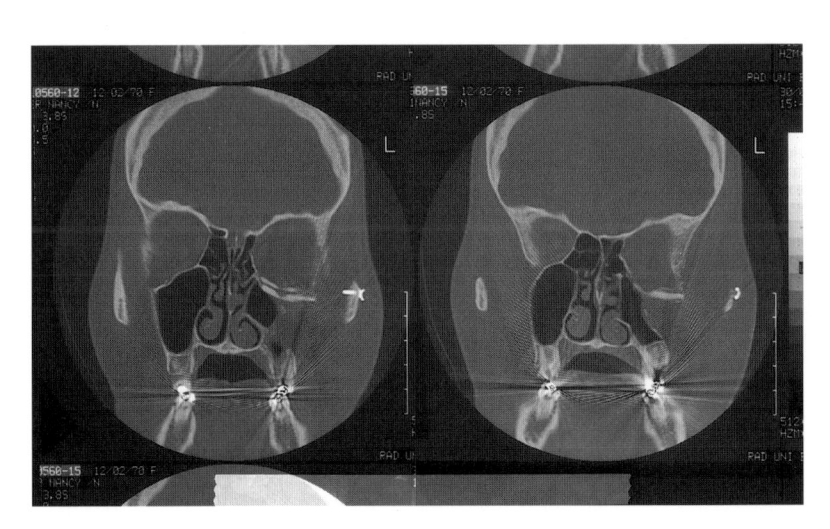

Figure 7.25. Technical error in orbital reconstruction. Enlargement of the posterior orbit from a dislocated bone graft. This type of defect requires the use of rigid fixation techniques.

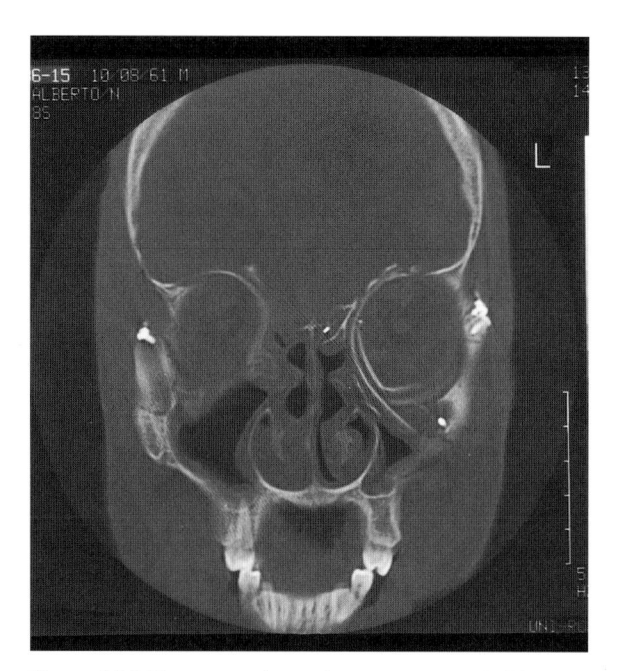

Figure 7.26. Not an error but no longer recommended. Reconstruction of a complex orbital wall defect with layered rib grafts. Secondary dislocation of one rib into the maxillary sinus.

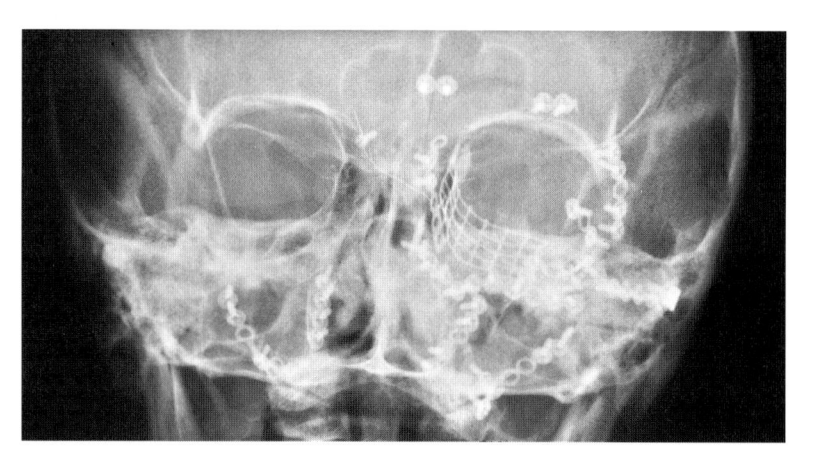

Figure 7.27. Error in the use of a titanium orbital plate. Attempt to reconstruct a two-wall defect with a large orbital plate. The plate is too short and produces constriction in the middle section of the orbit with posterior enlargement. The patient exhibits enophthalmos with a severe ocular motility disorder and double vision in the primary field of gaze.

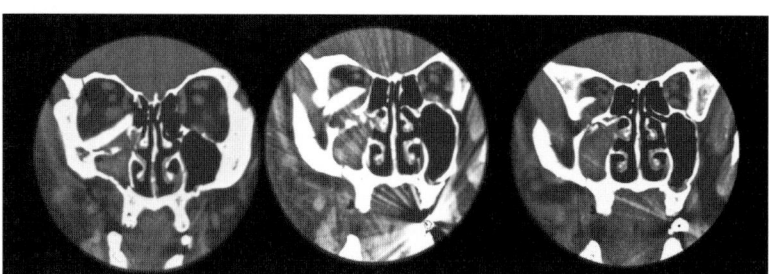

Figure 7.28. Error in the use of a rigid graft. A moderate sized orbital floor defect was bridged with a 3 x 2 cm calvarial bone graft. The graft protrudes into the deep orbit, resulting in severe eye motility disorder with double vision in the primary field of gaze. Comment: A rigid graft cannot be fitted to the complex orbital shape. In this case, it should have been wedged into the defect. Alternatively, a flexible graft could have been used for this relatively small defect.

Chapter 8
Secondary Corrections

Inadequate treatment of complex orbital fractures can result in severe deformities with significant functional and esthetic implications.

Typical sequelae of inadequately treated orbital fractures include enophthalmos, telecanthus and loss of malar prominence, the latter often combined with increased facial width.

Telecantus and loss of malar prominence are signs for an incorrectly reduced orbital frame, while enophthalmos ensues because of enlargement of the internal orbit.

The Soft Tissue Deformity

Healing of the inadequately supported soft tissues leads to shrinking, thickening, and malpositioning of landmarks. The resulting soft-tissue deformity creates special reconstructive difficulties.

Although the introduction of craniofacial techniques together with rigid fixation allows predictable and stable repositioning of malaligned facial fractures, surgeons dealing with secondary posttraumatic deformities know how frequently frustration results when they see the final outcome of a seemingly perfect bony correction. The reason for these limitations lies in the difficulty in dealing with traumatized and scarred soft tissue structures.

8.1 Principles of Corrective Surgery

There are two basic elements of corrective surgery:

- Reconstruction of the skeletal deformity
- Rearrangement of the soft tissue envelope with its landmarks.

Skeletal Reconstruction

The pattern of posttraumatic skeletal deformities is usually quite complex, with the gross dislocation of large fragments being responsible for significant deformities, while smaller fragments are associated with contour irregularities and distorted soft-tissue landmarks. Bone defects may also be related to resorption of bone fragments separated by soft tissues.

The goal of bony correction is the reestablishment of the pretraumatic skeletal anatomy. Often, it will not be possible to exactly duplicate the pretraumatic anatomy, and the reconstructive surgeon must seek a "skeletal balance" in order to achieve a harmonious external appearance. In orbito-zygomatic deformities, the adequate advancement of the zygoma and orbital rims depends on the degree of enophthalmos correction that can be achieved. Maximal advancement of the orbital ring may intensify the appearance of enophthalmos.

Grossly dislocated elements are refractured and reduced to an adequate position [3, 167]. Rigid fixation prevents recurrent late dislocation [116, 168, 169]. Minor contour irregularities are smoothed by grinding or with onlay bone grafts. Large implants for contour correction, especially in the malar area, are not recommended: Usually, it is difficult to blend the edges between a large onlay and the remaining skeleton, and we prefer to accept minor malpositioning of the segments.

Soft Tissue Rearrangement

Extensive avulsion of soft tissues may occur with the initial injury, with resultant healing in the wrong position. Displaced and improperly reduced bone fragments can also cause distortion of the soft tissue landmarks.

For proper correction, the soft tissues must be completely rearranged over the repositioned skeleton. This requires a degloving of the entire area involved in the initial trauma, with subsequent resuspension using subperiosteal face lift techniques [170, 171].

Multistage Correction

Correction of posttraumatic deformities usually requires several operative steps [98–100, 172], with different tactical approaches employed. While Yaremchuk prefers a single major correction followed by one or two "touch ups," Cohen et al. divide the skeletal correction into an outer (zygoma and LeFort I level) and inner part. We follow Yaremchuk's procedure, by performing the periorbital correction in one step. However, the "touch-up" procedures often become major repetitions of the previous surgery with significant improvement.

8.2 Diagnosis

Clinical examination is the most important element. Utilizing a combination of inspection, palpation, and measurements, the basic facial contours, dimensions and the position of important landmarks are noted. This includes sensory and motor nerve function testing.

Measurements include Hertel exophthalmometry (normal anterior projection of the globe 12–18 mm) and the intercanthal distance (normal range 30–34 mm).

Standardized photographs (face, eyes, worm's eye view) serve as a baseline for documentation and planning.

High-resolution computerized tomography in two planes permits in-depth analysis of the skeletal deformity. Three-dimensional (3D) reformatted CTs are illustrative and helpful for patient explanation. The axial and coronal scans continue to be indispensable for precise assessment of bony dislocations and orbital-wall defects.

We have used computer-generated 3D models for the planning of skeletal repositioning [173]. In certain situations it is helpful in clearly demonstrating the full extent of the skeletal dislocation. With experience, however, the use of 3D models becomes less important.

A preoperative ophthalmologic analysis is necessary to coordinate the treatment in patients with diplopia, as well as for medicolegal reasons.

8.3 Surgical Technique

Exposure

A combination of coronal, infraorbital, and upper buccal sulcus incisions is employed. The entire area involved in the initial trauma is subperiosteally reflected, which permits three-dimensional skeletal reconstruction and rearrangement of the soft tissues in the correct position. This approach cannot be overstressed.

The incisions are performed in the standard fashion. Incisions utilized for the primary repair must be taken into account and may require modifications in the approach.

The lower eyelid incision must be planned carefully. For secondary corrections, high subciliary incisions should be avoided, even if the primary access was done in this way. Often, there is already some degree of lower lid shortening from previous operations, which may become more pronounced with a subciliary approach. An incision in the lower third of the eyelid is recommended [163].

Exposure of the internal orbit is performed following the same guidelines as in primary reconstruction (see Chapter 7); scarring makes this a more difficult task. In areas with wall defects, there is a fusion between extraorbital tissues and the periorbit. The easiest method for determining the plane of cleavage is to begin by exposing as much of the uninjured orbit as possible, typically the supero-lateral quadrant.

In the orbital floor, care must be taken to preserve the infraorbital nerve, which is often embedded in scar tissue. The entire intraorbital dissection should be performed under loupe magnification.

Prior to and following dissection of the internal orbit, a forced duction test is performed, usually with some improvement after complete elevation of the periorbit. A significant difference compared to the uninjured orbit will remain because of scarring within the periorbit, with only a few cases showing no improvement at all. These patients often have a fixed deviation of an eye, signifying excessive intra-periorbital scarring. In these cases, the prognosis for cosmetic as well as functional improvement is very poor.

Figure 8.1 (a-d). Malrotation of the zygoma. The outward rotation creates a defect in the lateral orbital wall (a, b) as well as shortening and overbending of the zygomatic arch (c, d). >>>

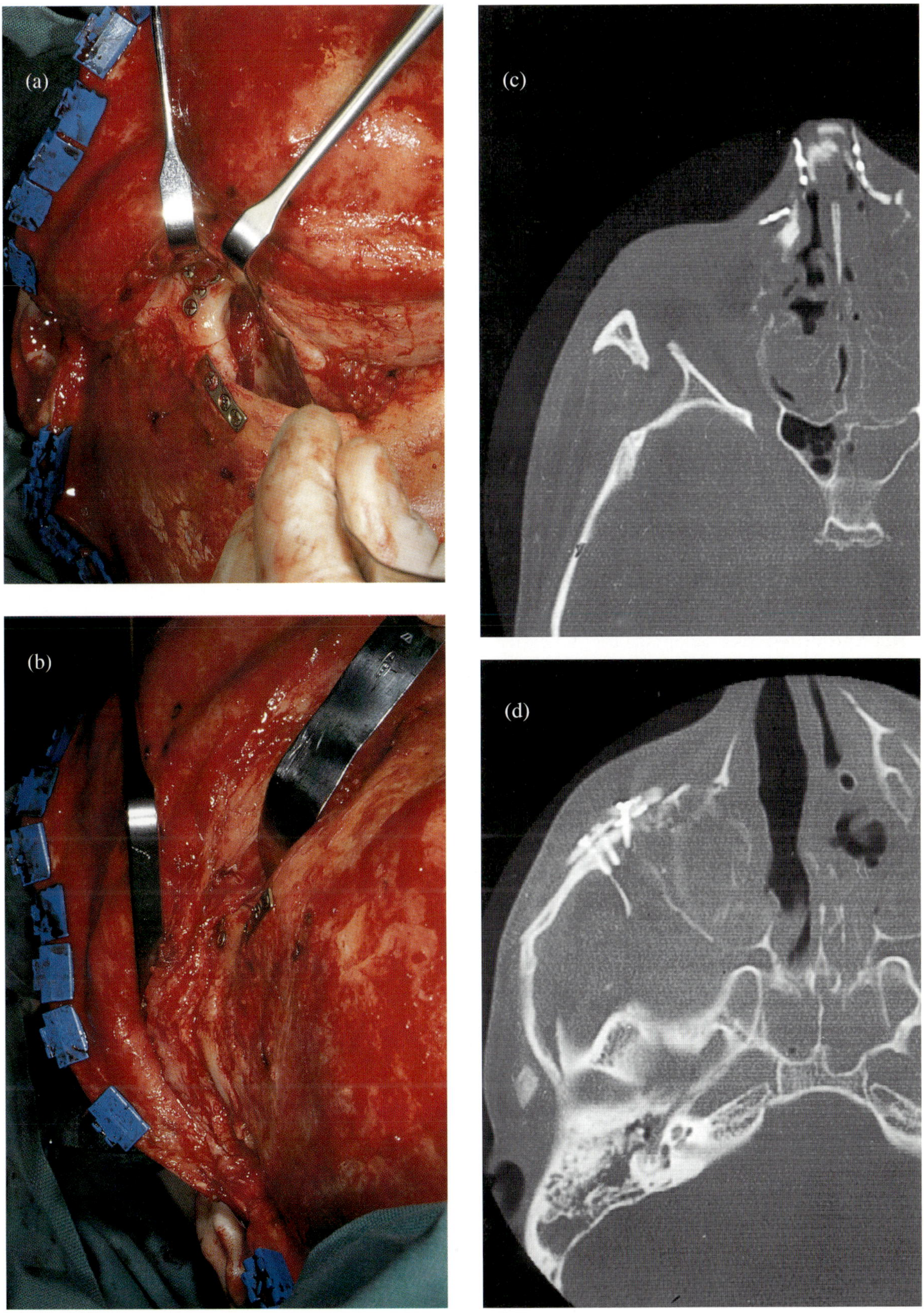
(a)
(b)
(c)
(d)

Skeletal Reconstruction

For the purposes of discussion, the orbit may be divided into four zones, which can treated separately: zygomatic, nasoethmoid, internal orbit, and orbital roof/supraorbital [100]. There are, of course, many injuries that affect several or all of these zones.

The sequence of skeletal reconstruction is the same as in primary repair, i.e. the first step is to reduce and stabilize the zygoma[11]. With the outer orbital frame as a reference, the remainder of the skeletal correction is then performed.

Zygomatic Complex

Malpositioning the zygoma typically leads to loss of malar prominence and increased facial width (Case 8.4). If a marked malrotation exists, the defect in the lateral orbital wall leads to orbital enlargement and enophthalmos [22].

After complete exposure of the zygomatic body, arch, and lateral orbital wall, the malpositioning can readily be identified (Figure 8.1). Often, there is only partial bony consolidation with interposed fibrous tissue. The initial fracture lines are recreated with saw and chisel, and where necessary, immature interpositional bone is removed. The correct position is determined with the help of the lateral orbital wall, allowing rigid fixation of the frontozygomatic suture with plates. This establishes the basic landmarks for subsequent reconstruction.

Minor malpositions of the zygoma without orbital enlargement are usually accepted.

Nasoethmoid Area

Deformities of the nasoethmoid area are difficult to correct for a variety of reasons. The unesthetic aspect of telecanthus is created not only by the in-

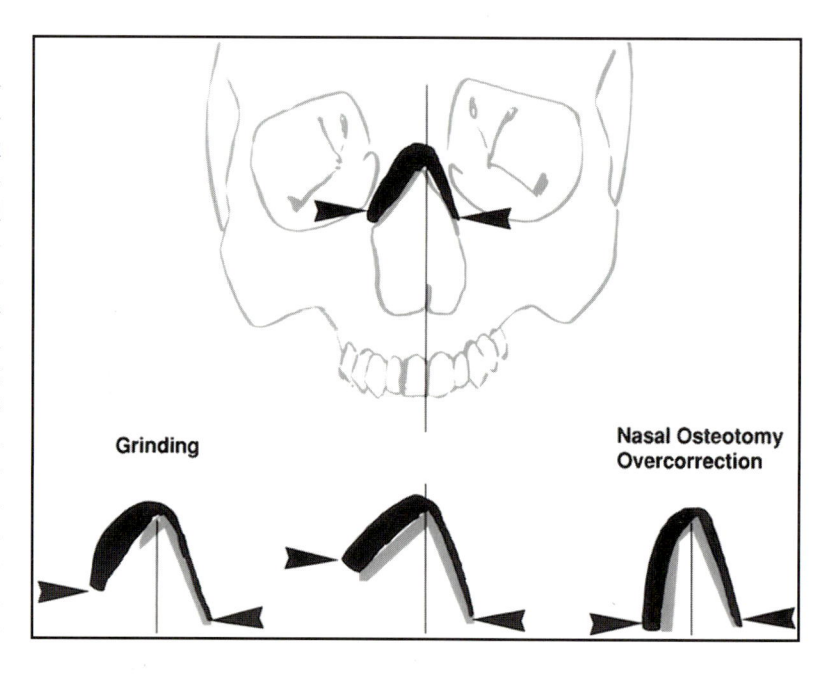

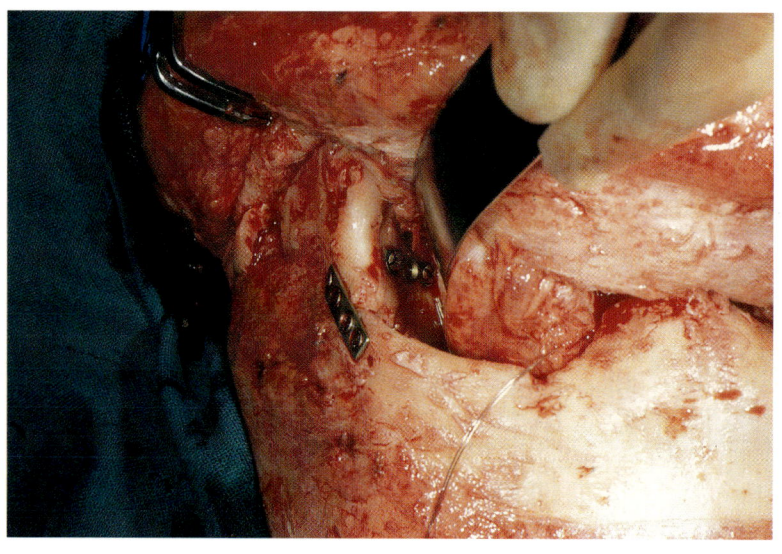

Figure 8.3. Geometry of telecanthus correction. Telecanthus is created by widening of the nasal base, usually with some degree of soft-tissue thickening. Adequate reduction of the intercanthal distance requires nasal osteotomy. With simple grinding, the nasal dorsum remains wide.

Figure 8.2. Reduction of zygoma. After reduction, the zygoma lines up correctly with the posterior part of the lateral orbital wall. The position of the zygoma has been secured with a plate inside the orbit (optional). Note the step between the reduced anterior part of the zygomatic arch and the root (arrow).

creased intercanthal distance, but also by the rounded palpebral fissure and the flattened nose. For correction, the entire nasal skeleton requires recontouring. This is accomplished with osteotomies of the nasal bones, including the lacrimal crest, and therefore the attachment of the inner canthal ligament. If the ligamentous insertion is still intact, it should be preserved because the normal anatomic configuration can never be perfectly imitated.

In this area, thickening of the soft tissues tends to compromise the result of the skeletal correction. Maximal skeletal narrowing should therefore be achieved in order to create a nearly normal intercanthal distance (Figure 8.3). Even with maximal narrowing, repair of telecanthus usually falls short of perfection [100].

Fixation of the mobilized nasal segments is performed using the same techniques as in primary repair. A transnasal wire secures the nasal bone fragment against outward rotation, even if a canthopexy is performed.

Medial Canthopexy

A detached medial canthal ligament is reduced with a separate transnasal canthopexy. The ligament is grasped with a 28-gauge wire at its origin, i.e. where the three limbs have not yet separated [142]. This wire is passed transnasally; the point of insertion must be above and behind the nasolacrimal duct. If the bone in this area does not permit creation of an insertion point, a miniplate can be used (Figures 8.4,

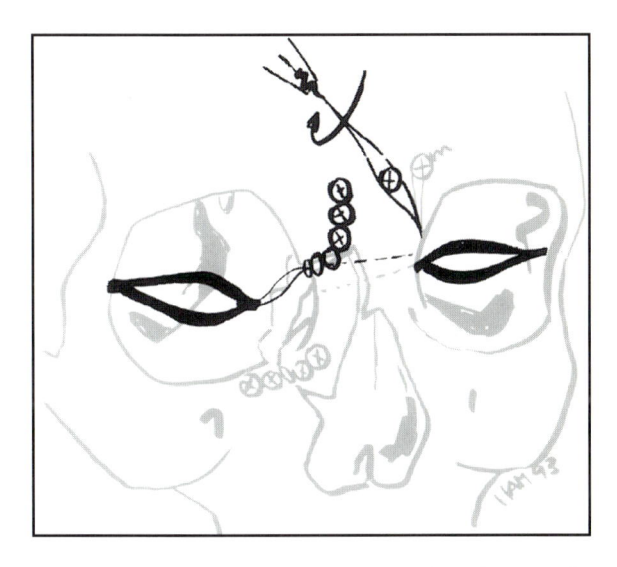

Figure 8.4. Nasal osteotomy and transnasal canthopexy. The nasal osteotomy is performed posteriorly to the lacrimal crest, with separate transnasal wires for the bone fragment and the canthal ligament. The insertion point for the canthal ligament can be created with a miniplate.

8.5). Tightening of the transnasal canthopexy is always the last step in secondary corrections prior to closure of the coronal flap. This is done because placement of bone grafts is facilitated by free canthal ligaments.

Nasal Bone Grafts

If augmentation of the nasal dorsum is necessary, this is done with an open rhinoplasty approach. A

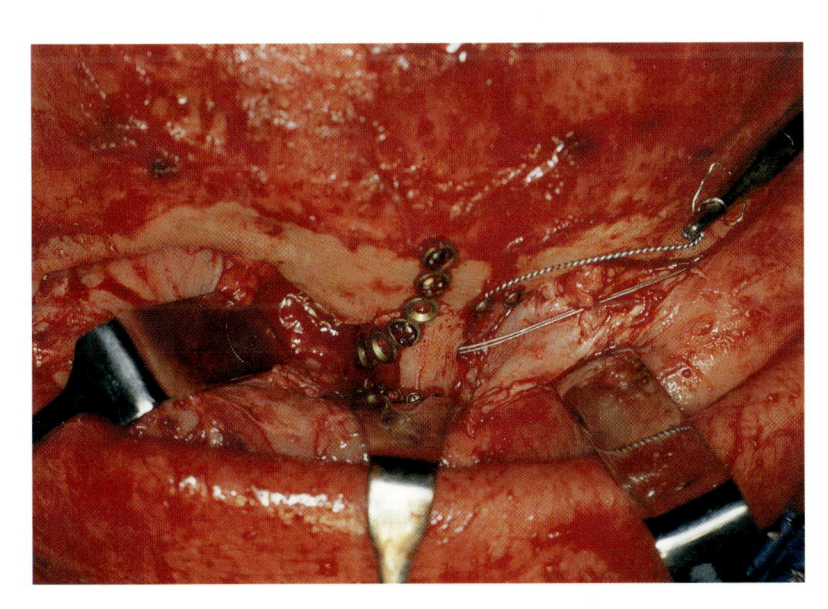

Figure 8.5. Intraoperative view. The nasal osteotomy has been performed, and overreduction of the bone is secured with a transnasal wire, which is already tightened. The canthopexy wire is left loose until bone grafting of the internal orbit is completed. Additional microplate for positioning of the nasal fragment.

split cranial bone graft is shaped, and the tip is placed between the medial crura of the alar cartilages in order to obtain a smooth contour [145].

Internal Orbit

The relation between enophthalmos and orbital volume and shape are discussed in detail in Chapter 2. Technical problems leading to inadequate reconstruction of the internal orbit are described in Chapter 6.

The aim of secondary reconstruction of the internal orbit is again the restoration of the preinjury shape and volume.

Complete circular dissection back into the posterior orbit is essential to expose the uninjured areas [15, 174]. Scarring may render the identification of stable posterior landmarks difficult.

There may be a real defect or merely a bony depression (Figure 8.6). Depending on this, rigid fixation techniques for the internal orbit or obliteration with bone or cartilage chips will be adequate. A forced duction test is performed before and after the insertion of bone grafts to detect eventual limitation of ocular motility by the grafts.

The grafts must be placed behind the axis of the globe, as bone grafts placed too anteriorly move the globe superior, not forward [175]. If possible, overcorrection in the antero-posterior direction is desirable during surgery, since it results in correct positioning after a few months. However, this is sometimes not possible, for the following reasons:

- Extensive scarring within the periorbit may be present. In these cases, even complete subperiosteal dissection far back into the posterior orbit provides only minimal anterior mobility.
- Scarring within the periorbit may be localized to one area. In this case, anterior mobilization is possible, but a deviation of the globe axis results [102]. Here, a compromise between anteroposterior position and rotational position must be sought.

- If there is severe scarring of the eyelids, anterior movement of the globe may prevent their complete closure. Again, a compromise between anterior projection and the danger of corneal desiccation must be found.

Orbital Roof/Supraorbital Region

In the supraorbital region, localized depressions or contour irregularities of the supraorbital rim may be corrected with onlay grafting.

Inferior displacement of the orbital roof leads to vertical globe dystopia and eventually to proptosis. Depending on the underlying skeletal deformity, correction may be done with or without craniotomy. In the former case, surgery should be carried out in cooperation with a neurosurgeon.

Soft Tissue Repositioning

After completion of the bony reconstruction, the soft tissues are redraped like a mask, with subperiosteal anchoring sutures used to suspend the cheek anteriorly and the SMAS laterally.

Temporal hollowing may be corrected by advancement of the temporal muscle, with complete mobilization necessary to permit adequate anterior rotation (Case 8.2).

An important element of soft-tissue repositioning lies in the correct placement of the canthal ligaments (placement of the medial canthal ligaments has been discussed previously). While the insertion of the medial canthal ligaments is preserved, if possible, the lateral ligaments are routinely detached during surgery and must be repositioned in a slightly overcorrected position. Detachment of the lateral canthal ligaments enhances visibility to a great extent and reinsertion is not as difficult as reinsertion of the medial ligament.

Minor corrections include scar revisions, local onlays, blepharoplasties, and rhinoplasties.

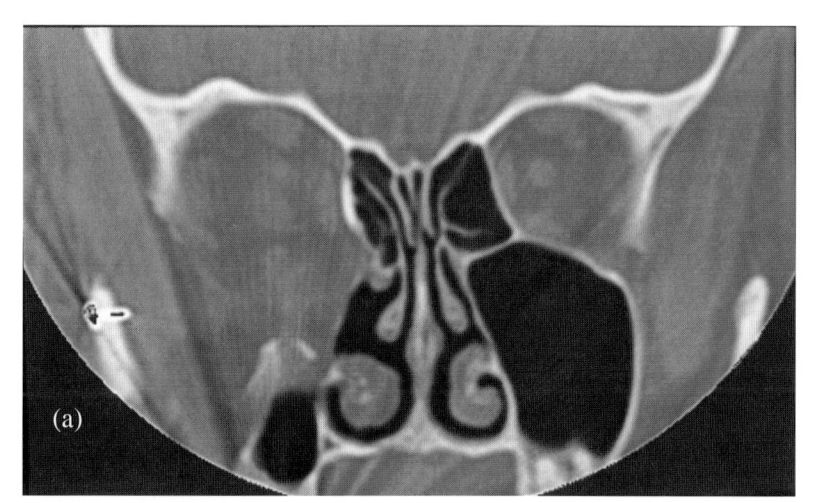

Figure 8.6 (a-d). Secondary reconstruction of the internal orbit. If a real defect is present (a), reconstruction is done with rigid fixation techniques for the internal orbit, as demonstrated in Chapter 7 (b). Often, there is merely a large depression (c), which is filled with bone or cartilage chips (d).

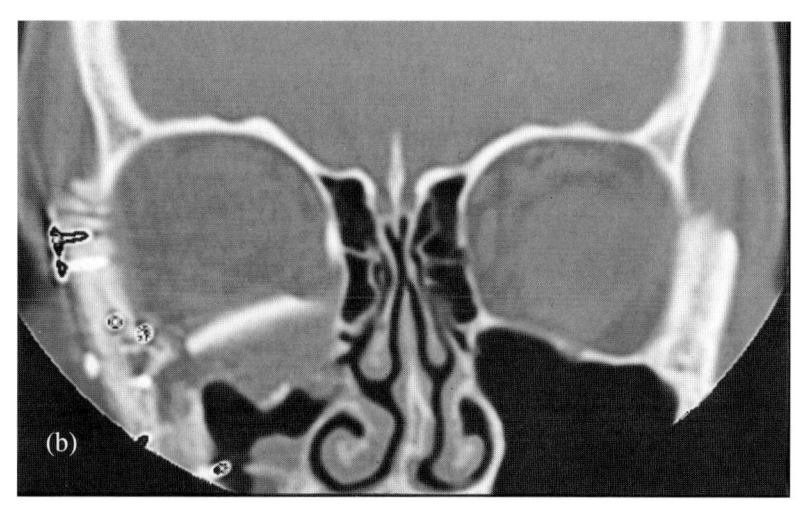

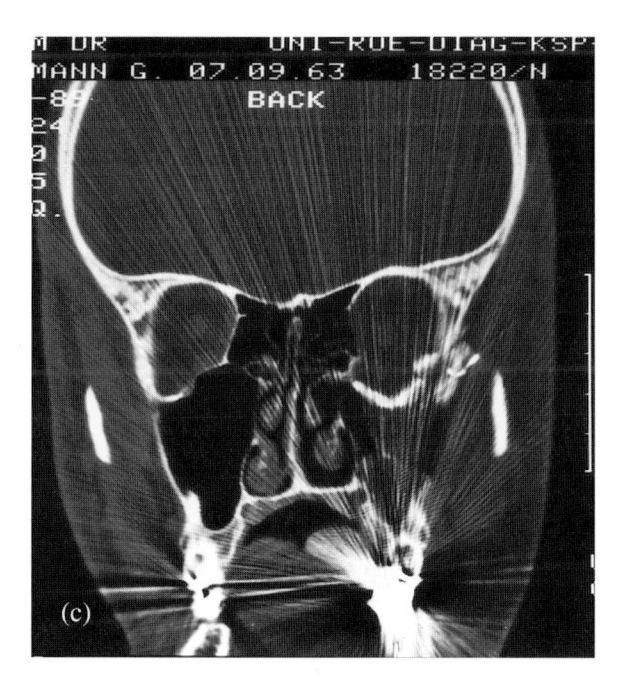

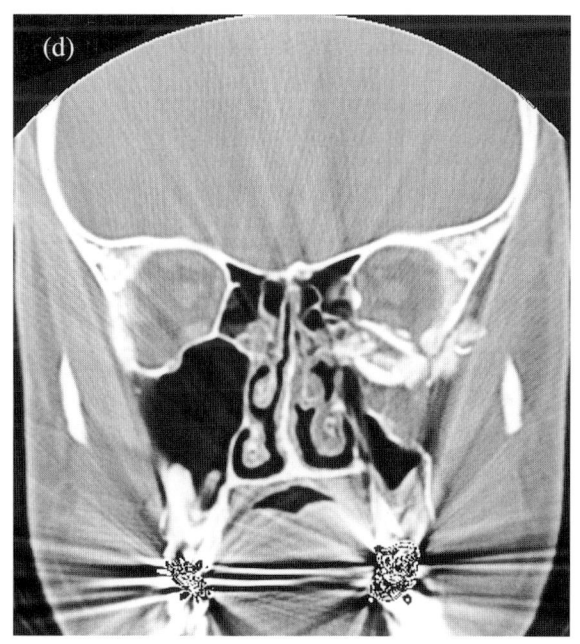

8.4 Complications

Secondary orbital reconstruction is not a benign procedure, and serious complications may be associated with this type of surgery [102, 176].

Ocular Complications

The most serious complication associated with secondary orbital reconstruction is visual impairment or blindness. Visual impairment has been reported by Iliff [102] and Tessier [177], and one of our own patients undergoing secondary orbital reconstruction sustained a complete loss of vision due to a bone fragment impinging on the optic nerve, despite subsequent decompression (see Section 6.2, Figure 6.7).

Infections

Because of scarring and decreased vascularity, the local resistance against infection is lower than in primary repair. Infection with subsequent extrusion of bone or alloplastic grafts from the orbit, the nose, or the cheek has been reported [98, 102]. In our patients, graft infection occurred, though 4 patients presented with orbital cellulitis originating from a frontal sinus infection. All these patients had had upper respiratory tract infection.

Other Complications

Other possible complications are frontal nerve damage, ectropion, or cerebral rhinorrhea.

8.5 Functional Aspects

Secondary corrections may influence binocular vision in a positive or negative sense, so functional aspects must be considered in planning surgical treatment.

Although enophthalmos is associated with diplopia in a high percentage of patients, this is not *always* the case; enophthalmos may occur without diplopia and vice versa.

Possible mechanisms leading to diplopia are discussed in Chapter 4.

If the patient has normal binocular vision, deterioration as a result of enophthalmos surgery is not very probable, although it is necessary to inform the patient about this possibility.

Different types and degrees of diplopia have different prognoses. Severely impaired ocular motility with a small but intact central field of vision may be a contraindication against enophthalmos surgery in light of the possible deterioration.

If diplopia is present, a careful ophthalmologic evaluation and coordinated planning is necessary, as it is important to discuss the rationale for secondary corrections very clearly with the patient and the ophthalmologist. Secondary orbital reconstruction per se often does not correct double vision. If only a minor degree of enophthalmos exists and diplopia is the only complaint, ophthalmologic therapy alone is sufficient. In severe deformities, however, orbital reconstruction should precede ocular muscle surgery for functional and esthetic reasons.

Sequence of Treatment

Before any ocular muscle surgery or injections, all reconstructive operations around the orbit must have been completed, including soft-tissue corrections, ligamentous insertions, and the eyelids.

The ophthalmologist should wait until no more spontaneous changes in eye motility and squint angle occur, as these could interfere with strabismus surgery. This usually requires 6–8 months.

8.6 Case Reports

Case 8.1 (Figure 8.7 a–d)
Telecanthus and Increased Facial Width

This 23-year-old patient was involved in a car accident and suffered multiple injuries including a panfacial fracture with rupture of the left globe, making enucleation necessary.

The skeletal deformity resulted from inadequate nasoethmoid and zygoma reduction and underbending of a plate stabilizing a fracture of the mandibular symphysis.

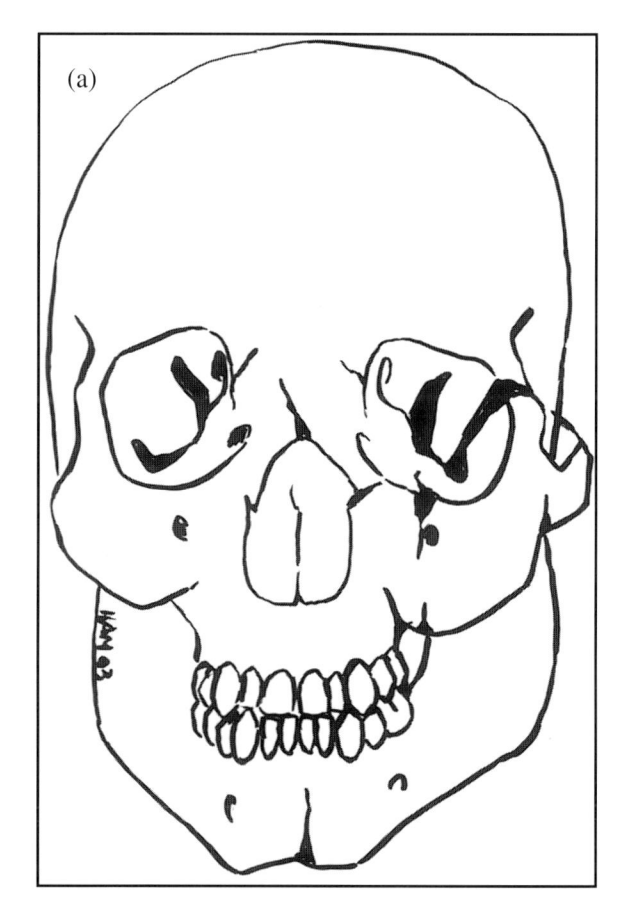

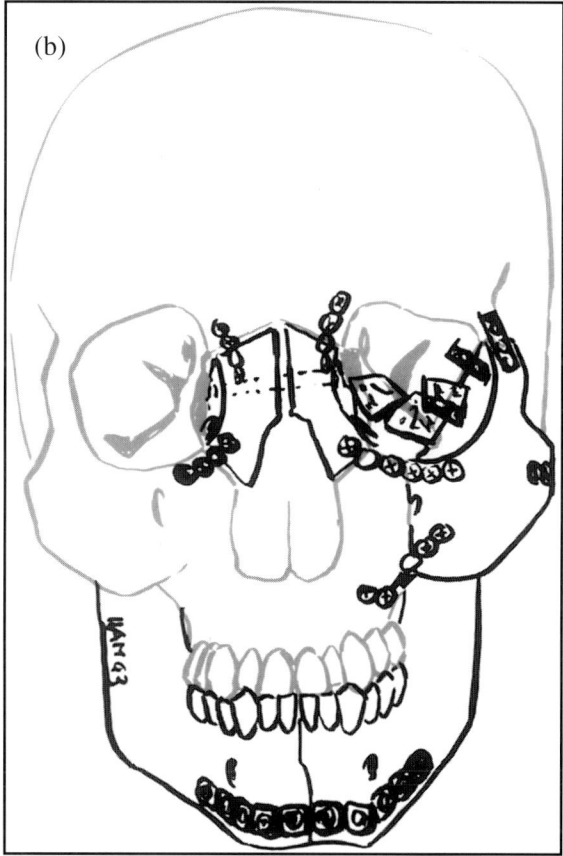

Figure 8.7 (a, b). Case 8.1: Skeletal deformity (a) and correction (b) in a patient after panfacial injury.

A schematic drawing is shown of the deformity (a) and the osteotomies performed during the first stage of correction (b). The patient is shown before (c) and 7 months after (d) two-stage correction. In a second correction, a segmental maxillary osteotomy and a genioplasty were performed.

Case 8.2 (Figure 8.8 a–d)
Complex Deformity of the Left Orbit

Complex deformity of the left orbit with telecanthus, enophthalmos and mild zygomatic deformity. The skeletal problem was aggravated by malpositioning of the lateral canthal ligament and temporal hollowing. The figure shows the skeletal deformity (a) and its correction with bilateral nasal osteotomies and bone grafting to the orbit (b). The zygomatic deformity was not addressed. Advancement of the temporal muscle corrected the temporal hollowing.

Case 8.3 (Figure 8.9 a–f)
Complex Posttraumatic Deformity of the Right Orbit

Complex posttraumatic deformity of the right orbit (a), with an intercanthal distance of 41 mm. Skeletal correction included nasal and zygomatic bone osteotomy as well as bone-graft reconstruction of the internal orbit (b). The patient is shown preoperatively (c) and 8 months after 4 stage correction (d). Despite repeated nasal osteotomy, the telecanthus was not entirely corrected. One possible reason may lie in soft tissue thickening resulting from a galeal flap used during the first correction to smoothen the irregular bony nasal skeleton. Enophthalmos (e) was not completely corrected (f).

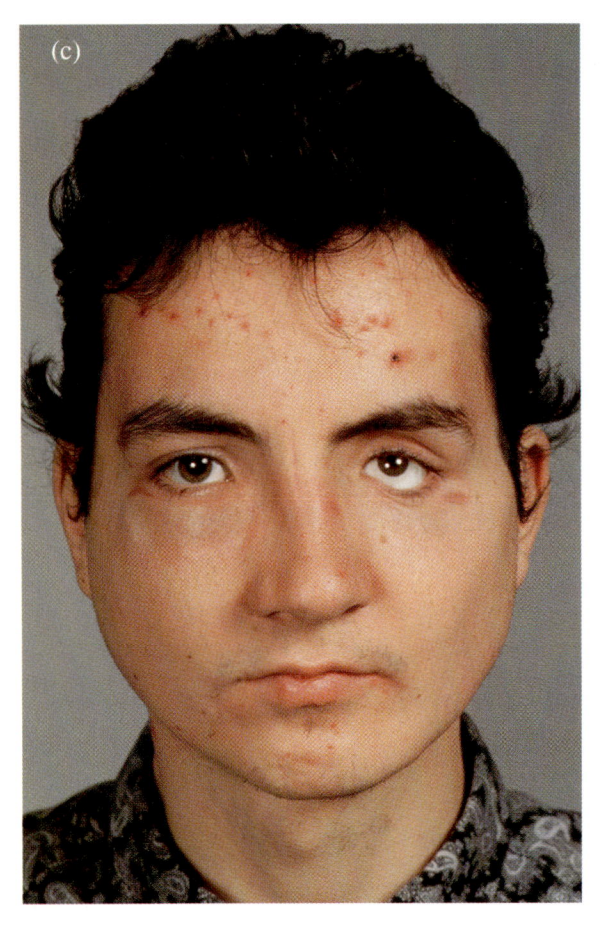

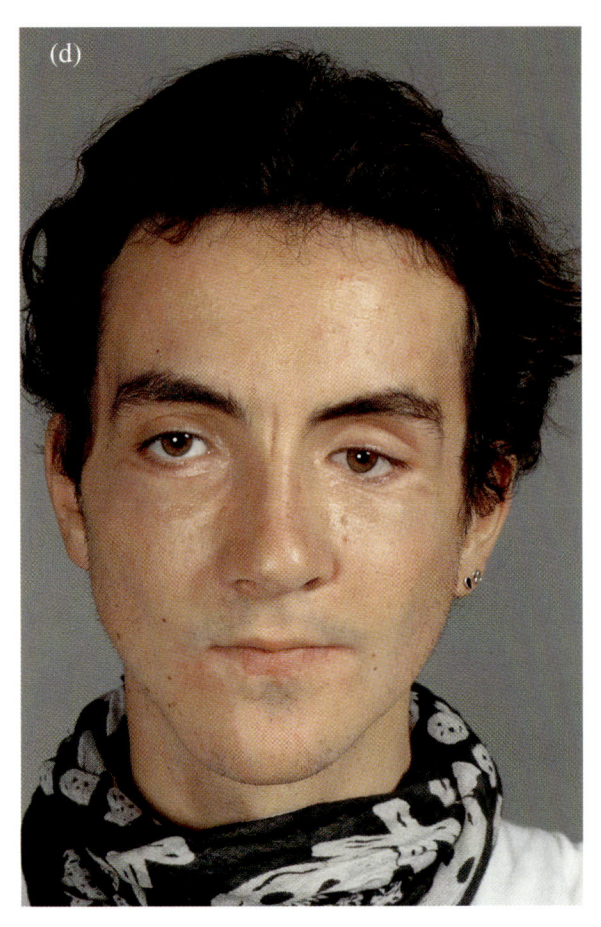

Figure 8.7 (c, d). Case 8.1: The patient before (c) and 7 months after two-stage correction (d).

Case No. 8.4 (Figure 8.10 a–g) Posttraumatic Deformity of the Right Orbit

Posttraumatic deformity of the right orbit with enophthalmos and malposition of zygoma (a). Corrective surgery included reosteotomy of the zygoma, orbital reconstruction, and transnasal medial canthopexy (b). The CT scan shows loss of malar prominence and increased facial width (c). The patient is shown prior to (d) and 9 months after two-stage correction (e). Reconstruction of the internal orbit was done using rigid fixation (see Figure 8.6 a, b).

Significant enophthalmos (f) was corrected (g).

Case No. 8.5 (Figure 8.11 a–d) Late Deformity after Orbital and Frontal Sinus Fracture

A depression of the orbital floor was present, while the main reason for the malposition of the eye was a large frontal mucocele (a). For correction, the mucocele was removed, and the depression in the orbital floor was filled with bone grafts (b). Patient is shown prior to (c) and 4 months after one-stage correction (d).

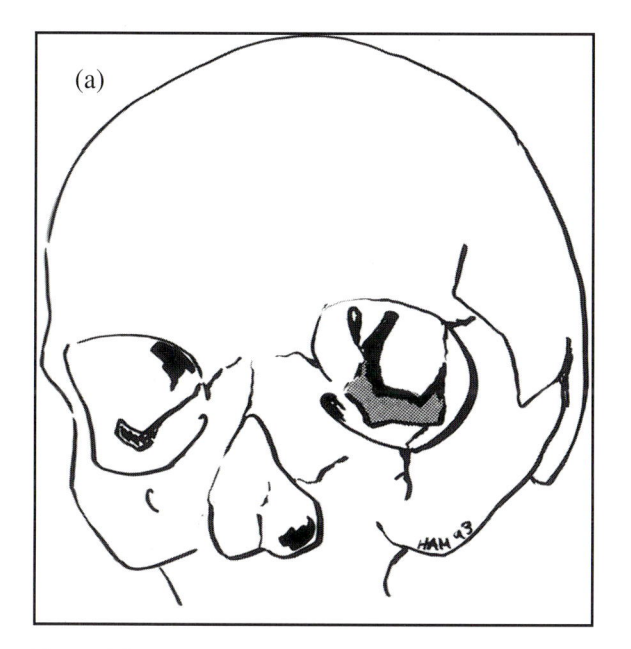

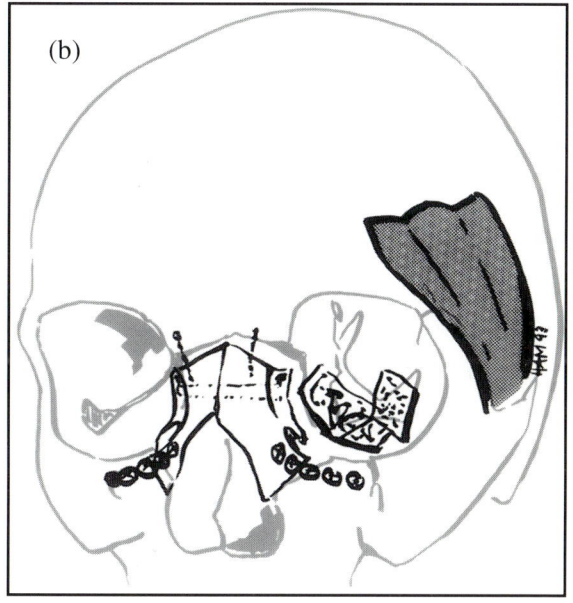

Figure 8.8 (a, b). Case 8.2: Complex posttraumatic deformity of the left orbit (a) with malpositioning of the nasal bones and defects in the orbital floor and medial wall. Skeletal correction included bilateral nasal osteotomies and bone grafting to the orbit. The temporalis muscle was advanced to compensate for temporal hollowing (b).

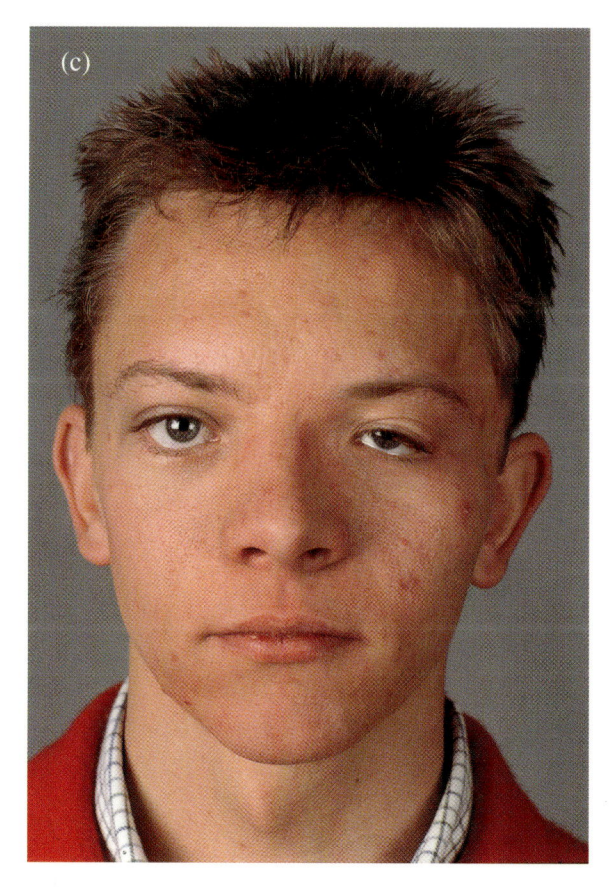

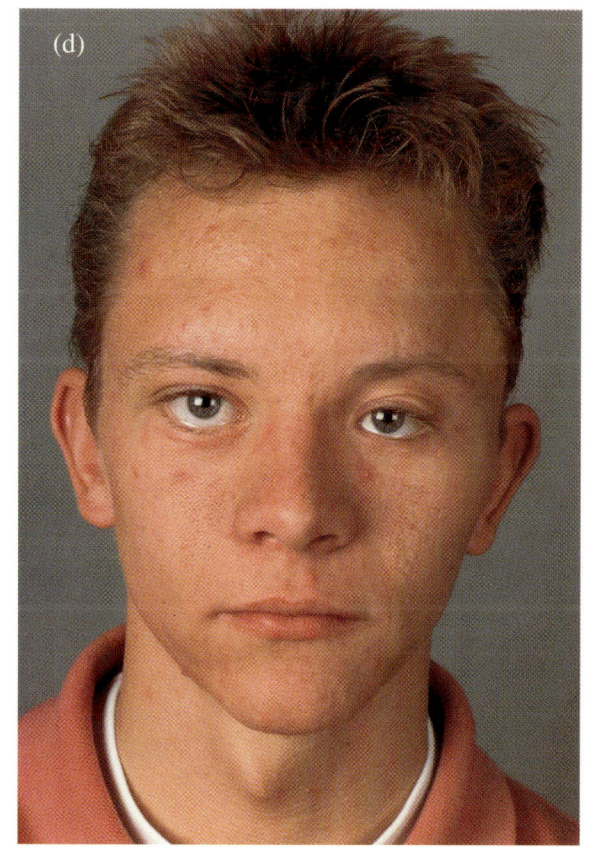

Figure 8.8 (c, d). Case 8.2: The patient before (c) and 6 months after one-stage correction (d).

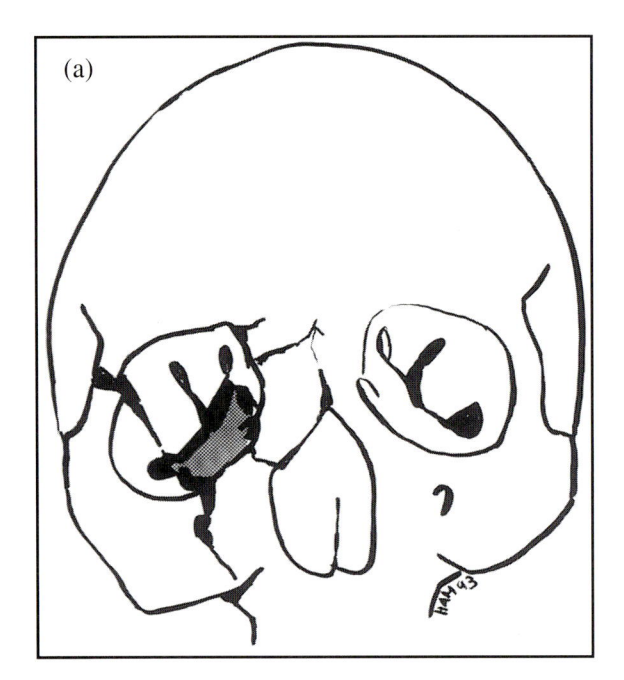

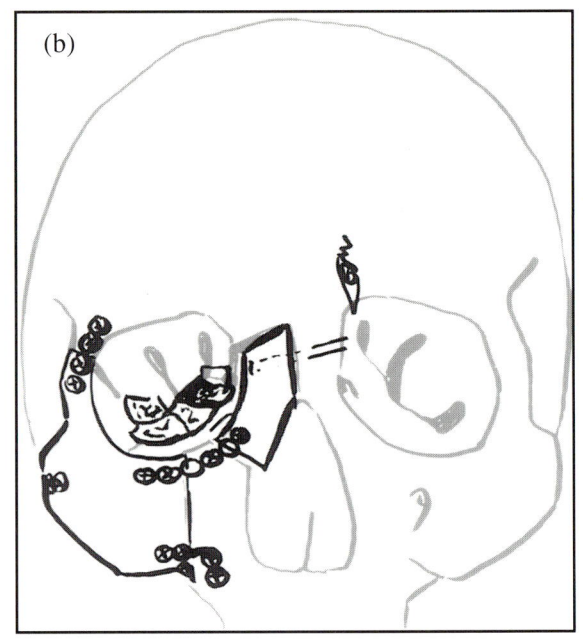

Figure 8.9 (a, b). Case 8.3: (a) Complex posttraumatic deformity of the right orbit with malpositioning of the zygoma, telecanthus, and defects of the orbital walls. (b) Skeletal correction included osteotomy of the zygoma and nasal osteotomy as well as bone grafting to the internal orbit.

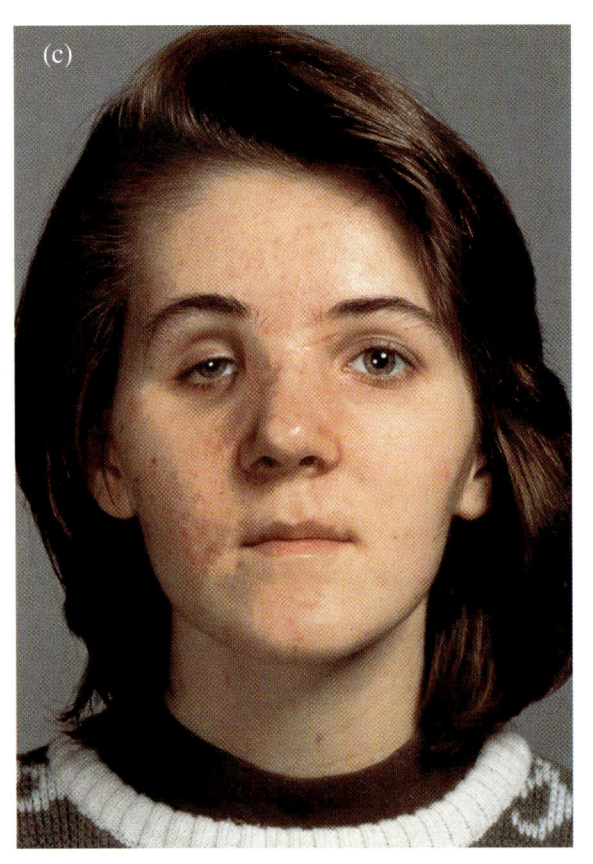

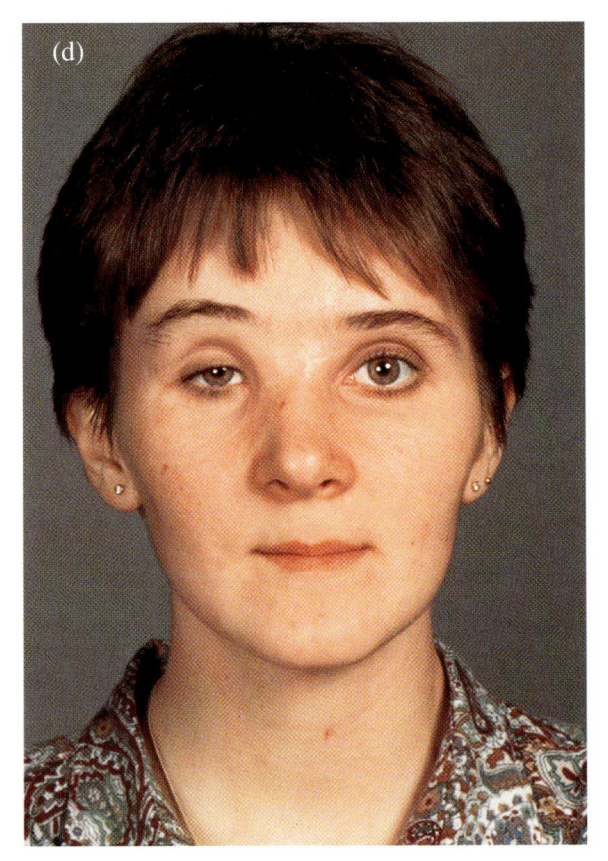

Figure 8.9 (c, d). Case 8.3: The patient before (c) and 8 months after four-stage reconstruction (d). Despite repeated nasal osteotomies, the appearance of telecanthus could not entirely be eliminated.

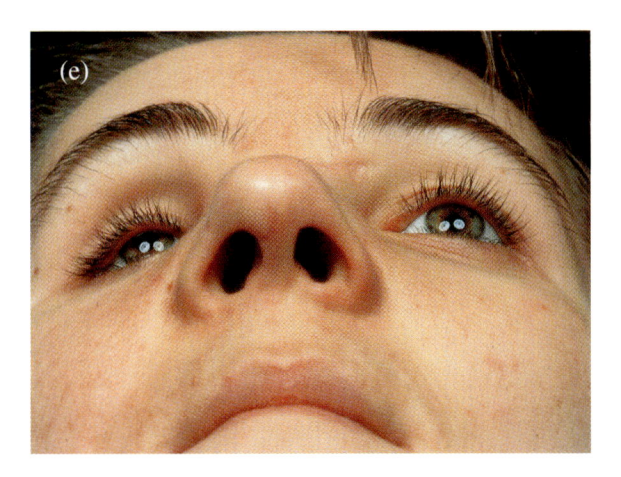

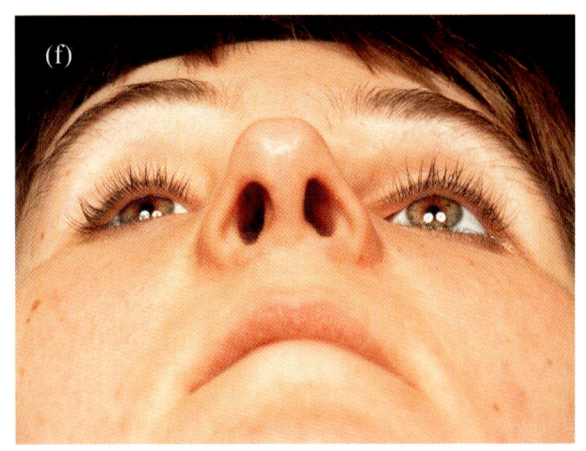

Figure 8.9 (e, f). Case 8.3: Significant enophthalmos (e) was partially corrected (f).

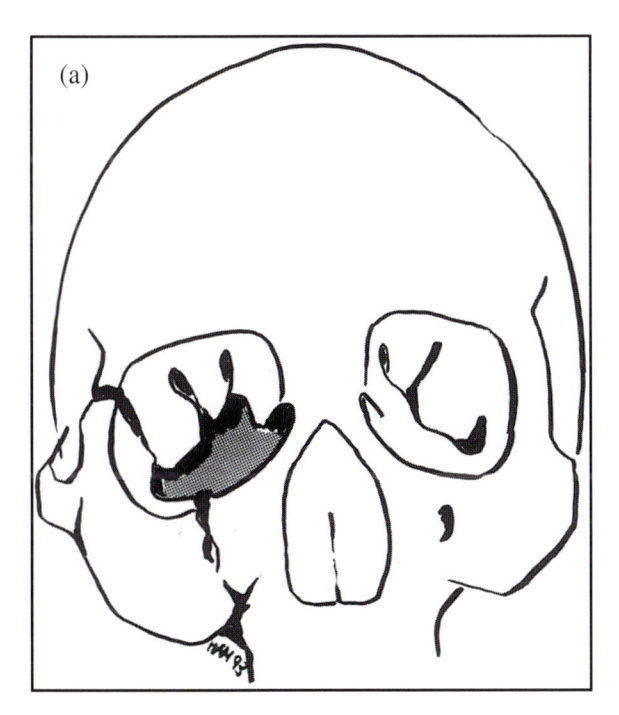

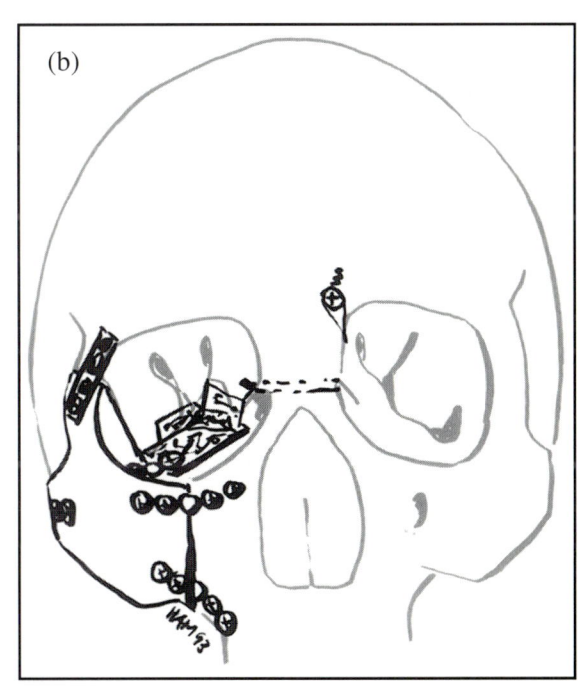

Figure 8.10 (a, b). Case 8.4: (a) Posttraumatic deformity of the right orbit with malpositioning of the zygoma, resulting in widening and shortening of the right hemiface. (b) Skeletal correction with osteotomy of the zygoma and bone grafting to the orbit.

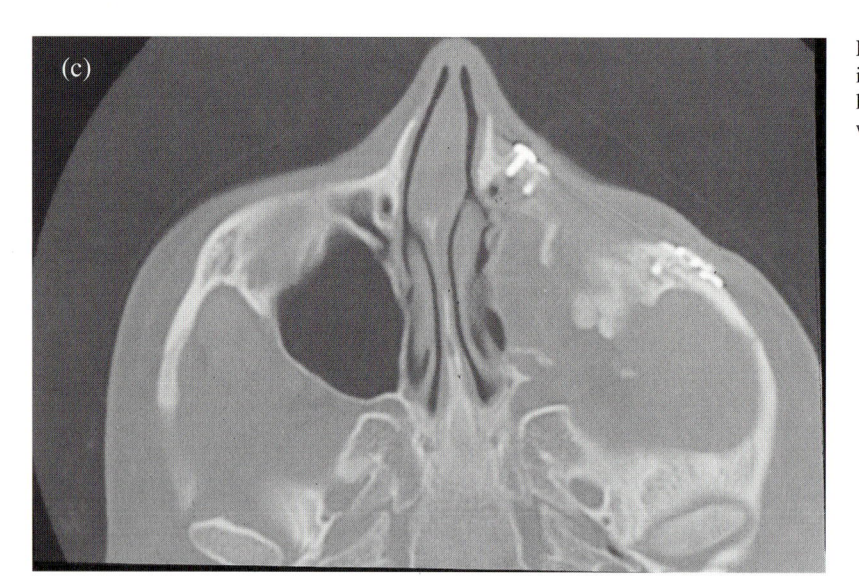

Figure 8.10 (c). Case 8.4: Malpositioning of the zygoma results in loss of malar prominence and increased facial width.

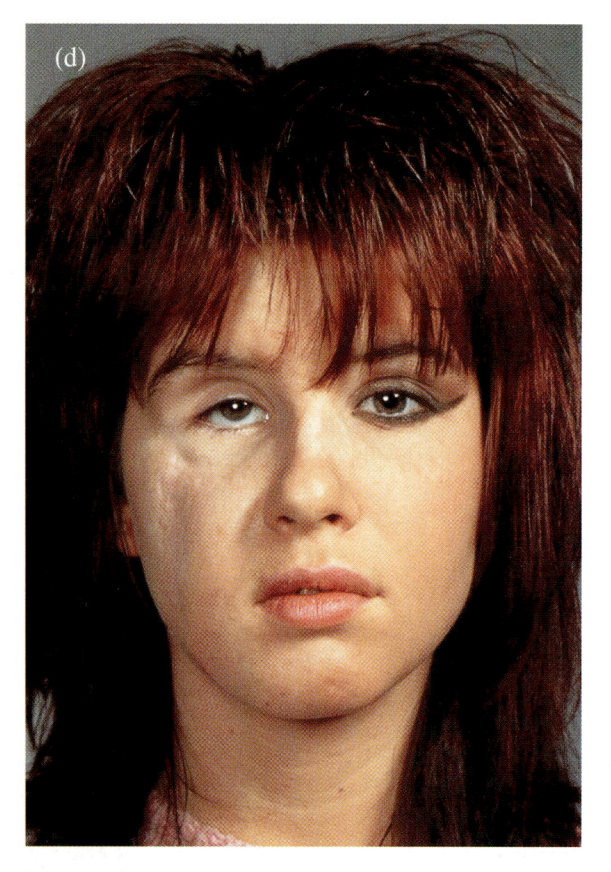

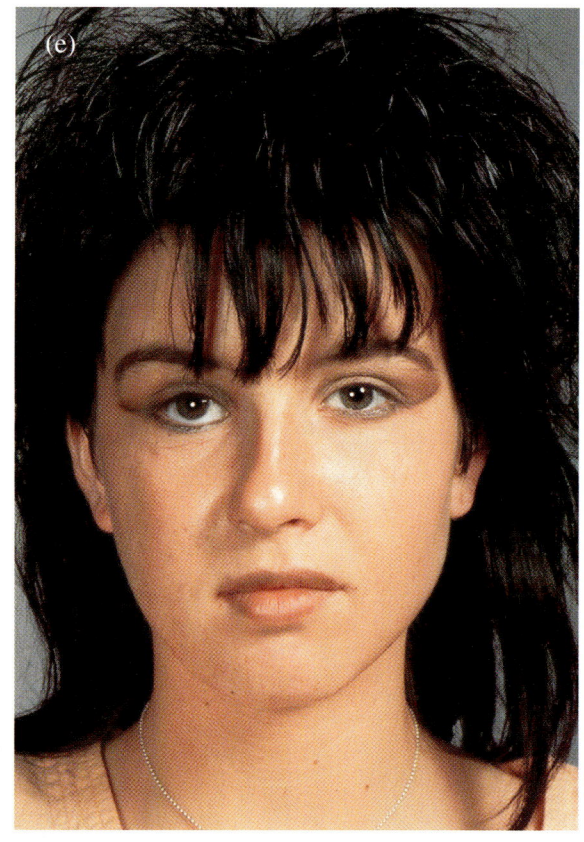

Figure 8.10 (d, e). Case 8.4: The patient before (d) and 9 months after two-stage correction (e).

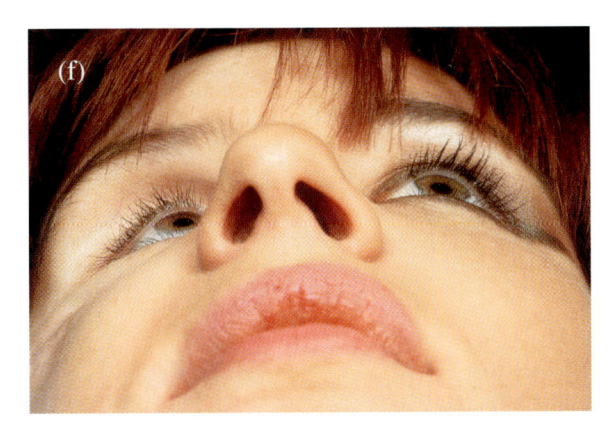

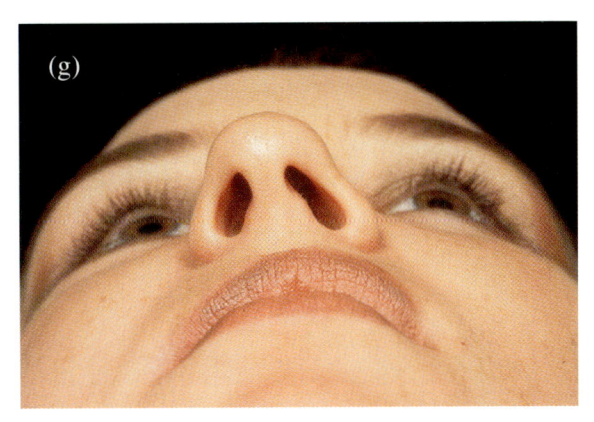

Figure 8.10 (f, g). Case 8.4: Significant enophthalmos (f) was corrected (g).

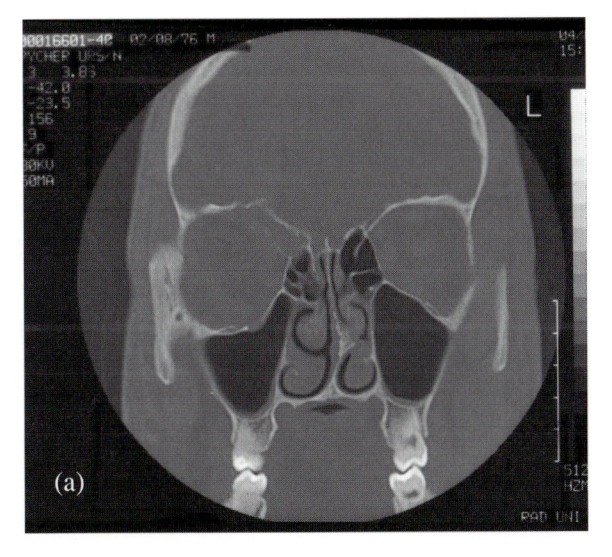

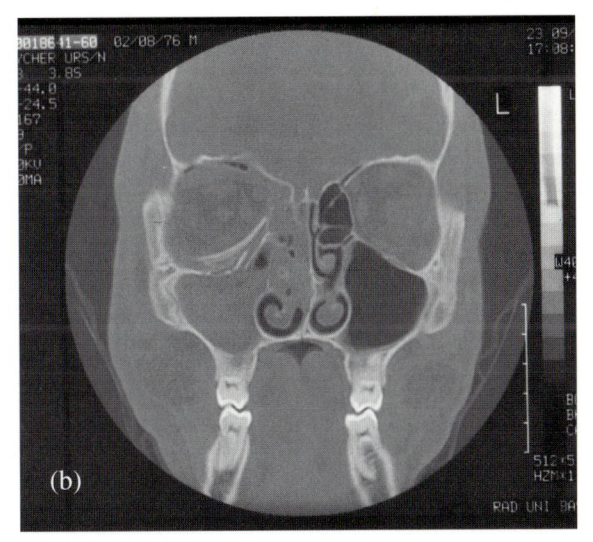

Figure 8.11 (a, b). Case 8.5: (a) Late posttraumatic deformity with vertical ocular dystopia due to mucocele of the right frontal sinus and depression of the orbital floor. (b) After removal of the mucocele and bone grafting to the orbital floor.

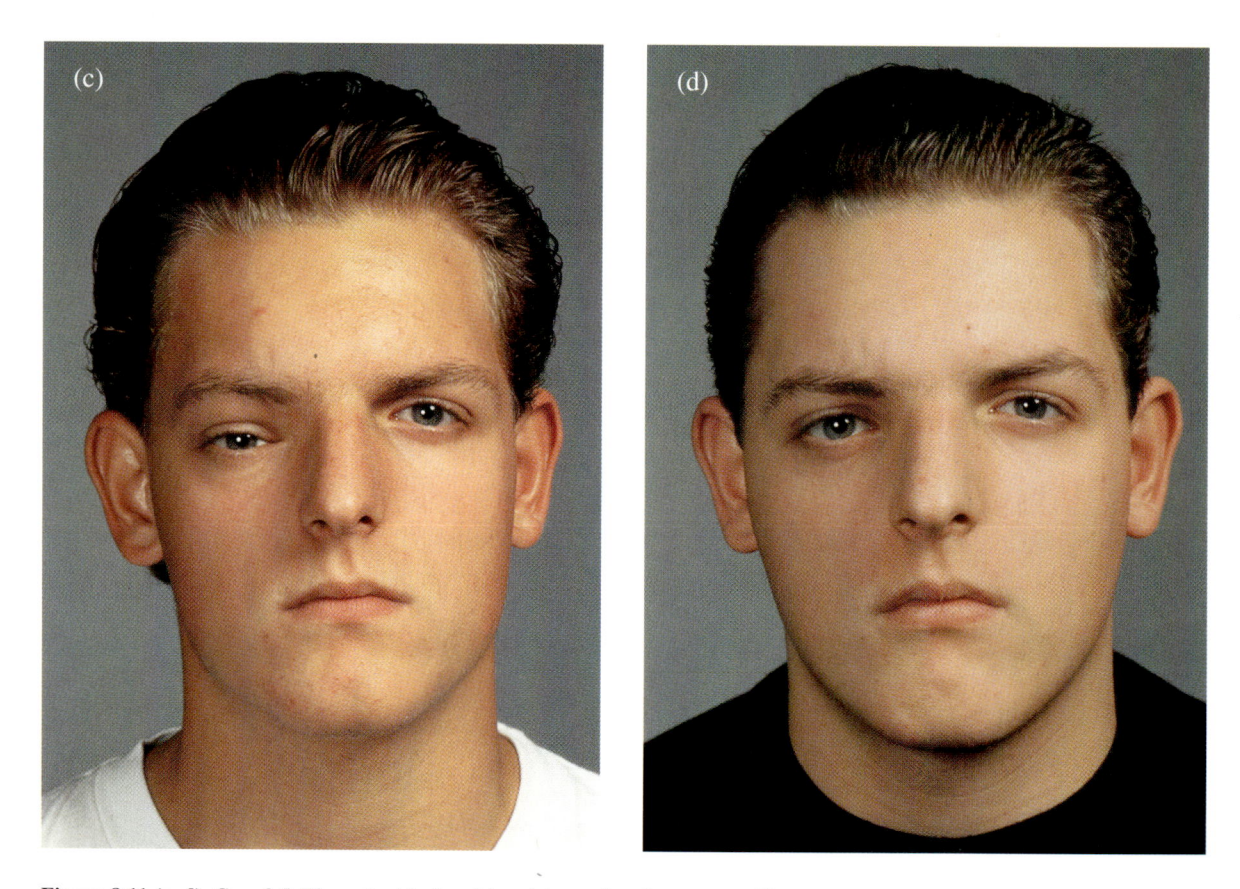

Figure 8.11 (c, d). Case 8.5: The patient before (c) and 4 months after surgery (d).

Chapter 9
Summary and Conclusion

This book has presented an overview of the diagnosis and treatment of orbital fractures, with particular emphasis on the surgical repair of complex injuries. Special chapters have dealt with the surgical anatomy of the orbit, the diagnosis of orbital fractures as well as ophthalmic aspects of orbital injuries.

As has been shown, for surgical purposes, the bony orbit may be divided into an orbital frame (orbital rim and zygoma) and the orbital walls. An area of special surgical interest lies in the posterior medial orbit: the key area. This area is of special importance in maintaining the antero-posterior position of the globe, and it must therefore be thoroughly reconstructed whenever involved in fractures.

The two important ophthalmic sequelae of orbital fractures are visual impairment and diplopia. Basic tests have been described which permit one to decide upon the necessity of consulting an ophthalmic surgeon.

A 5-year retrospective review of 448 patients with primary repair of orbital fractures constituted the database of the book. The most often encountered fractures are nonfragmented orbito-zygomatic fractures, constituting almost 75% of all orbital injuries.

Most of the fractures benefit from open reduction and rigid internal fixation with plates and screws, local incisions (lower eyelid and intraoral incisions) usually providing adequate exposure for reduction and stabilization. There is, however, a subgroup of fractures (20% of all orbital fractures), characterized by a major disruption of the orbital frame and/or significant orbital-wall defects, which require an extended exposure using a coronal approach as well as special reconstructive techniques. Identification and thorough treatment of these severe injuries is of utmost importance, inadequate management resulting in esthetic (enophthalmos, telecanthus, etc.) and functional (diplopia) sequelae that are very difficult to correct.

A critical review of 26 patients operated on for the above-mentioned sequelae has shown that esthetic and functional improvement may be achieved. However, the results always fall short of perfection, and serious complications may occur.

The initial treatment therefore must aim at a thorough restoration of the preinjury orbital shape and volume.

Endnotes

[1] In the literature, two controversial theories about the pathogenesis of blow-out fractures are discussed. The *hydraulic pressure theory* [30] suggests that a rise in intraorbital pressure causes the defect, whereas the *buckling force theory* [31] assumes it is caused by a force transmitted from the infraorbital rim. Isolated blow-out fractures are called "pure," whereas fractures associated with injuries to the orbital frame are called "impure" [32].

[2] Eye Hospital, Aarau, Switzerland.

[3] Ophthalmologic Clinic, University Hospital, Basel, Switzerland.

[4] The swinging flash light test (SFLT) is a very sensitive instrument in the diagnosis of optic nerve disfunction. To determine its accuracy, the second author (H.E. Killer, unpublished data) examined 67 patients with various optic neuropathies comparing the SFLT and visually evoked potentials (VEPs). Not a single false negative result was obtained compared to VEPs. We therefore conclude that VEPs are not necessary in the routine evaluation of acute traumatic visual impairment.

[5] The term "traumatic optic neuropathy" summarizes all extraocular, prechiasmatic pathologies leading to visual impairment. This includes retrobulbar and subperiosteal hematoma, blow-in fractures leading to reduced orbital volume, optic nerve sheath hematoma/edema, and direct injury to the nerve by bone fragments.

[6] The phenomena called "muscle sequelae" [83] consist of a sequence of events that start to develop if one eye muscle is not functioning properly. For example, if the left lateral muscle is paretic, the following events occur: (1) contracture of the ipsilateral antagonist (medial rectus) with secondary shrinking; (2) overfunction of the contralateral yoke muscle (right medial rectus); (3) secondary palsy of the contralateral antagonist.

[7] Five of the 513 patients with significant cerebral injuries died and were therefore excluded from the review.

[8] Optic nerve damage resulting in blindness complicated a secondary correction (see Table 7.2.8).

[9] The author is well aware of the shortcomings of such a rating. Yet would any other measurments be more appropriate to classify an esthetic result? The purpose of this classification was in fact more to force us to take a critical look at our results.

[10] The term "blow-out" signifies a *mechanism* rather than a given fracture pattern; thus, complex blow-out fractures may occur. It seems justifiable, however, to use the term in the generally accepted sense.

[11] Reconstruction of the supraorbital bar is closely related to the nasoethmoid reconstruction. A reconstructed anterior wall of the frontal sinus may interfere with canthopexy. This is the reason why we usually perform reconstruction of the supraorbital area after nasoethmoid repair has been done.

References

1. Ellis E, Attar A, Moos KF. An analysis of 2067 cases of zygomatico-orbital fractures. J. Oral Maxillofac. Surg. 1985; 43: 417–428.
2. Tessier P. The definitive plastic surgical treatment of the severe facial deformities of craniofacial dysostosis. Plast. Reconstr. Surg. 1971; 48(5): 419–441.
3. Tessier P. Total osteotomy of the middle third of the face for faciostenosis and for sequelae of Le Fort III fractures. Plast. Reconstr. Surg. 1971; 48: 533–541.
4. Tessier P, Gerard G, Derome P. Orbital hypertelorism. Scand J Plast Reconstr. Surg. 1973; 7: 39–58.
5. Gruss JS. Complex nasoethmoid-orbital and midfacial fractures: Role of craniofacial surgical techniques and immediate bone grafting. Ann. Plast. Surg. 1986; 17(5): 377–390.
6. Gruss JS, Bubak PJ, Egbert MA. Craniofacial fractures. An algorithm to optimize results. Clin. Plast. Surg. 1992; 19(1): 195–206.
7. Manson PN, Clifford CM, Su CT, Iliff NT, Morgan R. Mechanisms of global support and posttraumatic enophthalmos: I The anatomy of the ligament sling and its relation to intramuscular cone orbital fat. Plast. Reconstr. Surg. 1986; 77(2): 193–202.
8. Wolfe SA. Application of craniofacial surgical precepts in orbital reconstruction following trauma and tumour removal. J. Maxillofac. Surg. 1982; 10(4): 212–223.
9. Ochs MW, Buckley MJ. Anatomy of the orbit. Oral Max. Fac. Surg. Clin. North Am. 1993; 5(3): 419–429.
10. Montgomery Royce L. Head and neck anatomy with clinical correlations. New York: McGraw-Hill, 1981: 93–155.
11. Hollinshead W. Anatomy for surgeons (3rd ed.). Philadelphia: Harper & Row, 1982; vol. 1.
12. Lanz T. Orbita. In: Praktische Anatomie 1. Band: Kopf. Berlin, Heidelberg, New York: Springer, 1985.
13. Wolff E. Anatomy of the eye and orbit (6th ed.). Philadelphia: Saunders, 1968.
14. Manson PN, Hoopes JE, Su CT. Structural pillars of the facial skeleton: An approach to the management of Le Fort fractures. Plast. Reconstr. Surg. 1980; 66: 54–61.
15. Kawamoto HK. Late posttraumatic enophthalmos: a correctable deformity? Plast. Reconstr. Surg. 1982; 69: 423–430.
16. Manson PN, Glassman D, Iliff N, Vanderkolk C, Dufresne C. Rigid fixation of fractures of the internal orbit. Plast. Surg. Forum 1988; 11: 80–82.
17. Tessier. Personal communication. 1989.
18. Rontal E, Rontal M, Guilford FT. Surgical anatomy of the orbit. Ann. Otol. Rhinol. Laryngol. 1979; 88: 382–386.
19. Rootman J. Basic anatomic considerations. In: Rootman J, ed. Diseases of the orbit. Philadelphia: J. B. Lippincott, 1988: 3–18.
20. Grether NS, Hammer B, Prein J. Orbitavermessungen. Medical thesis, Basel, 1991.
21. Koorneef L. Spatial aspects of the orbital musculo-fibrous tissue in man. Amsterdam and Lisse: Swets and Zeitlinger, 1977
22. Pearl RM. Surgical management of volumetric changes in the bony orbit. Ann. Plast. Surg. 1987; 19: 349–358.
23. Pearl RM. Prevention of enophthalmos: a hypothesis. Ann. Plast. Surg. 1990; 25: 132–133.
24. Manson PN, Grivas A, Rosenbaum A, Vannier M, Zinreich J, Illif N. Studies on enophthalmos: II Measurement of orbital injuries and their treatment by quantitative computed tomography. Plast. Reconstr. Surg. 1986; 77(2): 203–214.
25. Jackson IT. Classification and treatment of orbitozygomatic and orbitoethmoid fractures. The place of bone grafting and plate fixation. Clin. Plast. Surg. 1989; 16(1): 77–91.
26. Knight JS, North JF. The classification of malar fractures: an analysis of displacement as a guide to treatment. Br. J. Plast. Surg. 1961; 13: 325–338.
27. Zingg M, Laedrach K, Chen J, et al. Classification and treatment of zygomatic fractures: a review of 1,025 cases. J. Oral Maxillofac. Surg. 1992; 50(8): 778–790.
28. Larsen OD, Thomson M. Zygomatic fractures: a simplified classification for practical use. Scand. J. Plast. Reconstr. Surg. 1978; 12: 55–58.
29. Markowitz BL, Manson PN, Sargent L, et al. Management of the medial canthal tendon in nasoethmoid orbital fractures: the importance of the central fragment in classification and treatment. Plast. Reconstr. Surg. 1991; 87(5): 843–853.
30. Smith B, Regan WF. Blow-out fracture of the orbit: mechanism and correction of internal orbital fracture. Am. J. Ophthalmol. 1957; 44: 733 (cited after Manson, 1991).
31. Fujino T. Experimental blow-out fracture of the orbit. Plast. Reconstr. Surg. 1974; 54: 81–82.
32. Smith B, Converse JM. Early treatment of orbital floor fractures. Trans. Am. Acad. Opthalmol. Otolaryngol. 1957; 61: 602 (cited after Manson, 1991).
33. Antonyshyn O, Gruss JS, Fossel EE. Blow-in fractures of the orbit. Plast. Reconstr. Surg. 1989; 84: 10–20.
34. Banks P. The superior orbital fissure syndrome. J. Oral Surg. 1968; 24: 455–.
35. Dufresne CR, Manson PN, Iliff NT. Early and late complications of orbital fractures. Semin. Ophthalmol. 1989; 4: 176–189.
36. Zachariades N. The superior orbital fissure syndrome. Report of a case and review of the literature. J. Oral Surg. 1982; 53: 237–240.

37. Acartürk S, Dalay C, Kivanc Ö, Varinli I. Orbital apex syndrome associated with fractures of the zygoma and orbital floor. Eur. J. Plast. Surg. 1993; 16: 67–69.
38. Paskert JP, Manson PN. The bimanual examination for assessing instability in naso-orbitoethmoidal injuries. Plast. Reconstr. Surg. 1989; 83(1): 165–167.
39. Bite U, Jackson IT, Forbes GS, Gehring DB. Orbital volume measurments in enophthalmos using three-dimensional CT imaging. Plast. Reconstr. Surg. 1985; 75: 502–507.
40. Ilankovan V, Hadley D, Moos K, el Attar A. A comparison of imaging techniques with surgical experience in orbital injuries – a prospective study. J. Cranio. Max. Fac. Surg. 1991; 19(8): 348–352.
41. Forrest CR, Lata AC, Marcuzzi DW, Bailey MH. The role of orbital ultrasound in the diagnosis of orbital fractures. Plast. Reconstr. Surg. 1993; 92(1): 28–34.
42. Yab K, Tajima S, Imai K. Clinical application of a solid three-dimensional model for orbital wall fractures. J. Cranio-Max. Fac. Surg. 1993; 21: 275–278.
43. Anderson R, Panje W, Gross G. Optic nerve blindness following blunt forehead trauma. Opthalmology 1982; 89: 445–455.
44. McCoy FJ, Chandler RF, Magnan CG, et al. An analysis of facial fractures and their complications. Plast. Reconstr. Surg. 1962; 29: 381–391.
45. Mong AJ, Gossman MD. A prospective analysis of the incidence of ocular injury in 283 consecutive facial fracture patients. Presented during residents day at University of Louisville Departement of Ophthalmology (cited after Gossman 1992), 1990.
46. Tschanz A, Hammer B, Prein J. Visusverlust bei Verletzungen der Orbita. Medical thesis, Basel, 1994.
47. Miller GR. Blindness developing a few days after a midfacial fracture. Plast. Reconstr. Surg. 1968; 42: 384–386.
48. Katz B, Herschler J, Brich DC. Orbital hemorrhage and prolonged blindness: a treatable posterior optic neuropathy. Br. J. Ophthalmol. 1983; 67: 549–553.
49. Kersten RC, Rice CD. Subperiosteal orbital hematoma: Visual recovery following delayed drainage. Ophthalmic Surg. 1987; 18: 423–427.
50. Ord RA, El Attar H. Acute retrobulbar hemorrhage complicating a malar fracture. J. Oral Maxillofac. Surg. 1982; 40: 234–236.
51. Raflo GT. Blow-in and blow-out fractures of the orbit. Ophthalmic Surg. 1984; 15: 114–119.
52. Maniscalco JE, Habal MB. Microanatomy of the optic canal. J. Neurosurg. 1978; 48: 402–406.
53. Spoor TC. Traumatic optic neuropathies. 1993: 79–90.
54. Thompson HS. Pupillary signs in the diagnosis of optic nerve disease. Trans. Opthalmol. Soc. UK 1977; 96: 377–381.
55. Burde RM. The swinging flash light test. In: Clinical decision making in neuro-ophthalmology. St. Louis, Baltimore, Boston: Mosby, 1992: 7–9.
56. De Juan E, Sternberg P, Michels RG. Penetrating ocular injuries: types of injuries and visual results. Ophthalmology 1983; 90(11): 1318–1322.
57. Wolin MJ, Lavin PJM. Spontaneous visual recovery from traumatic neuropathy after blunt head injury. Am. J. Ophthalmol. 1990; 109: 430–435.
58. Fukado Y. Results in 400 cases of the surgical decompression of the optic nerve. In: Streiff EB, ed. Modern problems in ophthalmology, vol. 14. Basel: S. Karger, 1975: 474–81.
59. Seiff SR. High-dose corticosteroids for treatment of vision loss due to indirect injury to the optic nerve. Ophthalmic Surg. 1990; 21: 389–395.
60. Bracken MB, Shepard MJ, Collins WF, et al. A randomized, controlled trial of methylprednisolone or naloxone in the treatment of acute spinal-cord injury. New Engl. J. Med. 1990; 322(20): 1405–1411.
61. Braughler JM, Hall ED. Current applications of "high-dose" steroid therapy for CNS injury. J. Neurosurg. 1985; 62: 806–810.
62. Kline LB, Morawetz RB, Swaid S. Indirect injury to the optic nerve. Neurosurgery 1984; 14: 756–764.
63. Spoor TC, Hartel WC, Lensink DB, Wilkinson MJ. Treatment of traumatic optic neuropathy with corticosteroids. Am. J. Ophthalmol. 1990; 110: 665–669.
64. Krauseñ AS, OguranJ. H., Burde RM. Emergency orbital decompression: a reprieve from blindness. Otolaryngol. Head Neck Surg. 1981; 89: 252–256.
65. Funk GF, Stanley RBJ, Becker TS. Reversible visual loss due to impacted lateral orbital wall fractures. Head Neck Surg. 1989; 11(4): 295–300.
66. Lipkin AF, Woodson GE, Miller RH. Visual loss due to orbital fracture: the role of early reduction. Arch. Otolaryngol. Head Neck Surg. 1987; 113: 81–83.
67. Mauriello JA, DeLuca J, Krieger A, Schulder M, Frohmann L. Management of traumatic optic neuropathy – a study of 23 patients. Br. J. Ophthalmol. 1992; 76: 349–352.
68. Guy J, Sherwood M, Day AL. Surgical treatment of progressive visual loss in traumatic optic neuropathy. J. Neurosurg. 1989; 70: 799–801.
69. Spoor TC, Mathog RH. Restoration of vision after optic canal decompression. Arch. Ophthalmol. 1986; 104: 804–806.
70. Kennerdell JS, Amsbaugh GA, Myers EN. Transantral-ethmoidal decompression of optic canal fracture. Arch. Ophthalmol. 1976; 94: 1040–1043.
71. Mann W, Rochels R, Bleier R. Mikrochirurgische endonasale Dekompression des N. opticus. Fortschr. Opthalmol. 1991; 88: 176–77.
72. Niho S, Yasuda K, Sato T, Sugita S, Murayama K, Ogino N. Decompression of the optic canal by the transethmoidal route. Am. J. Opthalmol. 1961; 51: 659–665.
73. Lederman IR. Loss of vision associated with surgical treatment of the zygomatic orbital floor fracture. Plast. Reconstr. Surg. 1981; 68: 94–98.
74. Nicholson DH, Gazak SV. Visual loss complicating repairs of orbital floor fractures. Arch. Ophthalmol. 1971; 86: 369–375.
75. Ord RA. Postoperative retrobulbar hemorrage and blindness complicating trauma surgery. Br. J. Oral Surg. 1981; 19: 202–207.
76. Koorneef L. New insights into the orbital connective tissue. Arch. Ophthalmol. 1977; 95: 1269–1273.
77. Koorneef L, Zonneveld FW. The role of direct multiplanar high resolution CT in the assessment and management of orbital trauma. Radiol. Clin. North Am. 1987; 25(4): 753–766.
78. Fujino T, Makino K. Entrapment mechanisms and ocular injury in orbital blow-out fractures. Plast. Reconstr. Surg. 1980; 65: 571–576.

79. Wieser D. Inkomitanzverhalten bei verschiedenen okulären Bewegungsstörungen. Klin. Mbl. Augenheilk. 1993; 202(5): 397–403.
80. Elston JS. Paralytic strabismus: the role of botulinum toxin. Br. J. Ophthalmol. 1985; 69: 891–896.
81. Murray ADN. Early botulinum toxin treatment of acute sixth nerve palsy. Eye 1991; 5: 45–47.
82. Metz HS. Treatment of unilateral acute sixth nerve palsy with Botulinum toxin. Am. J. Ophthalmol. 1991; 112: 381–384.
83. Glaser JS. Neuro-ophthalmology. Lippincott 1990: 44–45.
84. Killer HE. Poster shown at the European Strabismus Congress, Salzburg (Austria). 1993.
85. Converse JM, Smith B, Obear MB, Wood-Smith D. Orbital blow out fractures: a ten year survey. Plast. Reconstr. Surg. 1967; 39(1): 20–33.
86. Converse JM. Two plastic operations for repair of the orbit following severe trauma and extensive comminuted fracture. Arch. Ophthalmol. 1944; 31: 323.
87. Putterman AM, Stevens T, Urist MJ. Non-surgical management of blow-out fractures of the orbital floor. Am. J. Ophthalmol. 1974; 77: 232–239.
88. Manson PN, Iliff N. Management of blow-out fractures of the orbital floor. II. Early repair for selected injuries. Surg. Ophthalmol. 1991; 35(4): 280–92.
89. Derdyn C, Persing JA, Broaddus WC, Delashaw JB, Levine PA, Torner J. Craniofacial trauma: an assessment of risk related to the timing of surgery. Plast. Reconstr. Surg. 1990; 86: 238–245.
90. Balle V, Christensen PH, Greisen O, Jorgensen PS. Treatment of zygomatic fractures: a follow-up study of 105 patients. Clin. Otolaryngol. 1982; 7: 411–416.
91. Iizuka T, Mikkonen P, Paukku P, Lindqvist C. Reconstruction of orbital floor with polydioxanone plate. Int J. Oral Maxillofac. Surg. 1991; 20(2): 83–87.
92. Gordon S, McCrae H. Monocular blindness as a complication of the treatment of a malar fracture. Plast. Reconstr. Surg. 1950; 6: 228–32.
93. Demas PN, Braun TW. Infection associated with orbital subcutaneous emphysema. Oral Maxillofac. Surg. 1991; 1239–1242.
94. Silver HS, Fucci MJ, Flanagan JC, Lowry LD. Severe orbital infection as a complication of orbital fracture. Arch. Otolaryngol. Head Neck Surg. 1992; 118(8): 845–8.
95. Stuzin JM, Wagstrom L, Kawamoto H, Wolfe SA. Anatomy of the frontal branch of the facial nerve: the significance of the temporal fat pad. Plast. Reconstr. Surg. 1989; 83(2): 265–271.
96. Tessier P. Autogenous bone grafts taken from the calvarium for facial and cranial applications. Clin. Plast. Surg. 1982; 9: 531–538.
97. Tessier P. Inferior orbitotomy: a new approach to the orbital floor. Clin. Plast. Surg. 1982; 9: 569575.
98. Cohen SR, Kawamoto HK. Analysis and results of treatment of established posttraumatic facial deformities. Plast. Reconstr. Surg. 1992; 90(4): 574–584.
99. Whitaker LA, Yaremchuk MJ. Secondary reconstruction of posttraumatic orbital deformities. Ann Plast. Surg. 1990; 25(6): 440–449.
100. Yaremchuk MJ. Changing concepts in the management of secondary orbital deformities. Clin. Plast. Surg. 1992; 19(1): 113–124.
101. Lambrecht JT. 3D-technology in maxillofacial surgery. Berlin, Chicago, Tokyo: Quintessenz, in press.
102. Iliff NT. The ophthalmic implications of the correction of late enophthalmos following severe midfacial trauma. Trans. Am Ophthalmol. Soc. 1991; 89(477): 477–548.
103. Mathog RH, Hillstrom RP, Nesi FA. Surgical correction of enophthalmos and diplopia: a report of 38 cases. Arch. Otolaryngol. Head Neck Surg. 1989; 115: 169–178.
104. Monasterio FO, Rodriguez A, Benavides A. A simple method for the correction of enophthalmos. Clin. Plast. Surg. 1987; 14: 169–175.
105. Roncevic HL. Refracture of untreated fractures of the zygomatic bone. J. Max. Fac. Surg. 1983; 11: 252–256.
106. Tessier P. The conjunctival approach to the orbital floor and maxilla in congenital malformations and trauma. J. Max. Fac. Surg. 1973; 1: 3–8.
107. Bähr W, Bagambis FB, Schlegel G, Schilli W. Comparison of transcutaneous incisions used for exposure of the infraorbital rim and orbital floor: a retrospective study. Plast. Reconstr. Surg. 1992; 90(4): 585–591.
108. Holtman B, Wray RC, Little AG. A randomized comparison of four incisions for orbital fractures. Plast. Reconstr. Surg. 1981; 67: 731–737.
109. Manson PN, Ruas E, Iliff N, Yaremchuk M. Single eyelid incision for exposure of the zygomatic bone and orbital reconstruction. Plast. Reconstr. Surg. 1987; 79(1): 120–126.
110. Antonyshyn O, Gruss JS, Galbraith DJ, Hurwitz JJ. Complex orbital fractures: a critical analysis of immediate bone graft reconstruction. Ann. Plast. Surg. 1989; 22(3): 220–233.
111. Al-Kayat A, Bramley P. A modified pre-auricular approach to the temporomandibular joint and malar arch. Br. J. Oral Surg. 1979; 17: 91–103.
112. Raveh J, Vuillemin T, Sutter F. Subcranial management of 395 combined frontobasal-midface fractures. Arch. Otolaryngol. Head Neck Surg. 1988; 114: 1114–1122.
113. Farmand MF. Titanium 3D plating system. Leibinger 1991 3–17.
114. Marsh JL. The use of the Würzburg system to facilitate fixation in facial osteotomies. Clin. Plast. Surg. 1989; 16: 49–60.
115. Munro JR. The Luhr fixation system for the craniofacial skeleton. Clin. Plast. Surg. 1989; 16: 41–48.
116. Prein J, Hammer B. The new AO 2.0 titanium plate set in cranio-maxillofacial surgery. AO/ASIF Dialogue 1989; 11(1): 9–12.
117. Rudderman RH, Mullen RL. Biomechanics of the facial skeleton. Clin. Plast. Surg. 1992; 19(1): 11–29.
118. Greenberg A, Hammer B, Prein. J. Pancraniomaxillofacial fractures. In: Greenberg A, ed. Craniomaxillofacial fractures: Principles of internal fixation using the AO/ASIF technique. New York, Berlin, Heidelberg: Springer Verlag, 1993: 193–207.
119. Tengvall P, Elwing H, Sjoequist L, Lundstroem I, Bjursten LM. Interaction between hydrogen peroxide and titanium: a possible reason for the biocompatibility of titanium. Biomaterials 1989; 10(2): 118–120.
120. Perren SM, Pohler O. News from the lab: titanium as implant material. AO/ASIF Dialogue 1987; 1(3): 11–12.
121. Sullivan PK, Smith JF, Rozelle AA. Cranio-orbital reconstruction: safety and image quality of metallic implants on

CT and MRI imaging. Plast. Reconstr. Surg. 1994; in press.
122. Antonyshyn O, Gruss JS. Complex orbital trauma: the role of rigid fixation and primary bone grafting. Adv. Ophthalmic Plast. Reconstr. Surg. 1987; 7: 61–92.
123. Phillips JH, Rahn BA. Fixation effects on membranous and endochondral bone graft resorption. Plast. Reconstr. Surg. 1988; 82(6): 872–77.
124. Nguyen PN, Sullivan P. Advances in the management of orbital fractures. Clin. Plast. Surg. 1992; 19(1): 87–98.
125. Frodel JLJ, Marentette LJ, Quatela VC, Weinstein GS. Calvarial bone graft harvest. Techniques, considerations, and morbidity. Arch. Otolaryngol. Head Neck Surg. 1993; 119(1): 17–23.
126. Pensler J, McCarthy JG. The calvarial donor site: an anatomic study in cadavers. Plast. Reconstr. Surg. 1985; 75(5): 648–651.
127. Finkle DR, Kawamoto HK. Complications of harvesting cranial bone grafts. Presented at the 64th Annual Meeting of the American Association of Plastic Surgeons. Coronado, 1985.
128. Young VL, Schuster RH, Harris LW. Intracerebral hematoma complicating split calvarial bone-graft harvesting. Plast. Reconstr. Surg. 1990; 86(4): 763–765.
129. Phillips JH, Gruss JS, Wells MD, Chollet A. Periosteal suspension of the lower eyelid and cheek following subciliary exposure of facial fractures. Plast. Reconstr. Surg. 1991; 88(1): 145–148.
130. Altonen M, Kohonen A, Dickhoff K. Treatment of zygomatic fractures: internal wiring – antral packing – reposition without fixation. J. Maxillo. Fac. Surg. 1976; 4: 107–115.
131. Champy M, Galach KL, Kahn JL, Pape HD. Treatment of zygomatic bone fractures. In: Hjorting-Hansen, ed. Oral and maxillofacial surgery: Maxillofacial surgery. Proceedings from the 8th International Conference on Oral and Maxillofacial Surgery. Chicago: Quintessence Publishing, 1985.
132. Chuong R, Kaban LB. Fractures of the zygomatic complex. J. Oral Maxillofac. Surg. 1986; 44: 283–288.
133. Davidson J, Nickerson D, Nickerson B, Eng P. Zygomatic fractures: comparison of methods of internal fixation. Plast. Reconstr. Surg. 1990; 86(1): 25–32.
134. Eisele DW, Duckert LG. Single-point stabilization of zygomatic fractures with the minicompression plate. Arch. Otolaryngol. Head Neck Surg. 1987; 113(3): 267–270.
135. Matsunaga RS, Simpson W, Toffel PH. Simplified protocol for treatment of malar complex fractures. Facial Plast. Surg. 1988; 5: 269–274.
136. Rohrich RJ, Hollier LH, Watumull D. Optimizing the management of orbitozygomatic fractures. Clin. Plast. Surg. 1992; 19(1): 149–65.
137. Rinehart GC, Marsh JL, Hemmer KM, Bresina S. Internal fixation of malar fractures: An experimental biophysical study. Plast. Reconstr. Surg. 1989; 84(1): 21–28.
138. Manson PN. Discussion of: Internal fixation of malar fractures: an experimental study, by Rinehart GC et al. Plast. Reconstr. Surg. 1989; 84(1): 26–27.
139. Prein J. Discussion of: Internal fixation of malar fractures: an experimental study, by Rinehart GC et al. Plast. Reconstr. Surg. 1989; 84(1): 28–29.
140. Gruss JS, Van Wyck L, Phillips JH, Antonyshyn O. The importance of the zygomatic arch in complex midfacial fracture repair and correction of posttraumatic orbitozygomatic deformities. Plast. Reconstr. Surg. 1990; 85(6): 878–90.
141. Stanley RB. The zygomatic arch as a guide to reconstruction of comminuted malar fractures. Arch. Otolaryngol. Head Neck Surg. 1989; 115: 1459–1462.
142. Zide BM, McCarthy JG. The medial canthus revisited – an anatomical basis for canthopexy. Ann. Plast. Surg. 1983; 11(1): 1–9.
143. Shore JW, Rubin PA, Bilyk JR. Repair of telecanthus by anterior fixation of cantilevered miniplates. Ophthalmology 1992; 99(7): 1133–1138.
144. Pollock RA. Nasal trauma. Pathomechanics and surgical management of acute injuries. Clin. Plast. Surg. 1992; 19(1): 133–147.
145. Leipziger LS, Manson PN. Nasoethmoid orbital fractures. Current concepts and management principles. Clin. Plast. Surg. 1992; 19(1): 167–193.
146. Romo T3, Jablonski RD. Nasal reconstruction using split calvarial grafts. Otolaryngol. Head Neck Surg. 1992; 107(5): 622–30.
147. Stanley RBJ. Management of frontal sinus fractures. Facial Plast. Surg. 1988; 5(3): 231–235.
148. Morain WD, Colby ED, Stauffer ME, Russell CL, Astorian DG. Reconstruction of orbital wall fenestrations with polyglactin 910 film. Plast. Reconstr. Surg. 1987; 80(6): 769–774.
149. Polley JW, Ringler SL. The use of Teflon in orbital floor reconstruction following blunt facial trauma: a 20-year experience. Plast. Reconstr. Surg. 1987; 79(1): 39–43.
150. Rubin LR. Polyethylene as a bone and cartilage substitute: a 32 year retrospective. In: Rubin LR, ed. Biomaterials in reconstructive surgery. St. Louis: Mosby, 1982.
151. Rozema FR, Bos RR, Pennings AJ, Jansen HW. Poly(L-lactide) implants in repair of defects of the orbital floor: an animal study. J. Oral Maxillofac. Surg. 1990; 48(12): 1305–1309.
152. Hendler BH, Gataeno J, Smith BM. Use of auricular cartilage in the repair of orbital floor defects. Oral Surg. Oral Med Oral Pathol 1992; 74(6): 719–722.
153. Höltje WJ. (Reconstruction of orbital floor defects with polyglactin). In: Pfeiffer G, Schwenzer N, ed. Fortschritte der Kiefer- und Gesichtschirurgie, vol. 28. Stuttgart: Thieme, 1983: 675–678.
154. De Sutter E, Dhooghe P, Baert C. Marlex mesh in the reconstruction of blow-out fractures of the orbit. Bull. Soc. Belge Ophtalmol. 1988; 228.
155. Ilankovan V, Jackson IT. Experience in the use of calvarial bone grafts in orbital reconstruction. Br J. Oral Maxillofac. Surg. 1992; 30(2): 92–96.
156. Waite PD, Clanton JT. Orbital floor reconstruction with lyophilized dura. J. Oral Maxillofac. Surg. 1988; 46(9): 727–730.
157. Berhaus A. Porous polyethylene in reconstructive head and neck surgery. Arch. Otolaryngol. Head Neck Surg. 1985; 111: 154–160.
158. Tessier. 1986 (cited after Nguyen 1992).
159. Sewall SR, Pernoud FG, Pernoud MJ. Late reaction to silicone following reconstruction of an orbital floor fracture. J. Oral Maxillofac. Surg. 1986; 44(10): 821–825.
160. Jordan DR, Onge PS, Anderson RL, Patrinely JR, Nerad JA. Complications associated with alloplastic implants used

in orbital fracture repair. Ophthalmology 1992; 99: 1600–1608.
161. Fenske NA, Vasey FB. Silicone-associated connective-tissue disease. The debate rages (editorial comment). Arch. Dermatol. 1993; 129(1): 97–98.
162. Silver RM, Sahn EE, Allen JA, et al. Demonstration of silicon in sites of connective-tissue disease in patients with silicone-gel breast implants. Arch. Dermatol 1993; 129(1): 63–68.
163. Wolfe SA. Posttraumatic orbital deformities. In: Wolfe SA, Berkowitz S, ed. Plastic surgery of the facial skeleton. Boston/Toronto: Little, Brown and Company, 1989: 575–623.
164. Glassman RD, Manson PN, Petty P, Vanderkolk C, Iliff N. Techniques for improved visibility and lid protection in orbital explorations. J. Craniofac. Surg. 1990; 1(1): 69–71.
165. Sullivan PK, Rosenstein DA, Holmes RE, Craig D, Manson PN. Bone graft reconstruction of the monkey orbital floor with iliac grafts and titanium mesh plates: a histometric study. Plast. Reconstr. Surg. 1993; 91(5): 769–775.
166. Phillips JH. Discussion of: Bone graft reconstruction of the monkey orbital floor with iliac grafts and titanium mesh plates: a histometric study by Sullivan et al. Plast. Reconstr. Surg. 1993; 91(5): 776–777.
167. Wolfe SA. Treatment of posttraumatic orbital deformities. Semin. Ophthalmol. 1989; 4(3): 161–175.
168. Prein J, Schilli W, Hammer B, Reuther J, Sindet-Pedersen S. Rigid fixation of facial fractures. In: Fonseca RJ, Walker RV, ed. Oral and maxillofacial trauma, vol. 2. Philadelphia: W.B. Saunders Company, 1991: 1172–1232.
169. Schilli W, Ewers R, Niederdellmann H. Bone fixation with screws and plates in the maxillofacial region. Int. J. Oral Surg. 1981; 10/Suppl. (1): 329–332.
170. Ramirez OM, Maillard GF, Musolas A. The extended subperiosteal face lift: a definitive soft-tissue remodeling for facial rejuvenation. Plast. Reconstr. Surg. 1991; 88(2): 227–236.
171. Tessier P. Face lifting and frontal rhytidectomy. In: Ely JF, ed. Seventh International Congress of Plastic and Reconstructive Surgery. Rio de Janeiro, 1980 (cited after Ramirez 1991).
172. Freihofer HP, Van Damme PA. Secondary posttraumatic periorbital surgery. J. Cranio-Max. Fac. Surg. 1987; 15: 183–187.
173. Jacob AL, Hammer B, Niegel G, et al. First experience in the use of stereolithography in medicine. In: Chartoff RP, Lightman AJ, Schenk JA, ed. The Fourth International Conference on Rapid Prototyping. Dayton: University of Dayton, 1993: 121–133.
174. Manson PN, Ruas EJ, Iliff NT. Deep orbital reconstruction for correction of posttraumatic enophthalmos. Clin. Plast. Surg. 1987; 14: 113–121.
175. Pearl RM. Treatment of enophthalmos. Clin. Plast. Surg. 1992; 19(1): 99–111.
176. Manson PN. Personal communication. 1990.
177. Tessier P. Personal communication. 1991.

Subject Index

A
Age distribution 31
Algorithm
    for management of diplopia 27
    for management of visual loss 22
Anterior ethmoid artery 58
AO craniofacial system 47
Associated injuries 33

B
Blindness (see Visual loss)
Blow-in fractures
    definition 11
    visual loss and 18
Blow-out fractures
    definition 11
    treatment 54
Bone grafts (see Calvarial bone)
Botulinum toxin 28

C
Calvarial bone
    harvesting technique 47
    utilization 34, 55ff.
Canthopexy
    medial 77
    lateral 48, 78
Causes of fractures 32
Central fragment
    definition 8
    management 52
Closed reduction, of orbito-zygomatic
    fractures 49
Corneal light reflex 26
Coronal incision, technique 44f.
Corticosteroids, in treatment of visual loss 22
CT examination, indications 14

D
Decompressive surgery, indications 22
Diplopia
    frequency 39
    management 27
    mechanisms 24f.

E
Ectropion 36
Electromyography 27
Enophthalmos
    anatomic basis 5f.
    correction 38
    diagnostic relevance 78
    frequency 38
Eye muscle surgery
    types 28
    timing 80

F
Face lift techniques (see Soft tissue resuspension)
Follow-up protocol 35
Forced duction test 26
Fracture patterns 32f.
Frontal nerve
    injury 44
    preservation 45
Frontal sinus injuries 53f.

G
Globe injuries 18, 39
Grafting, of orbital wall defects
    frequency 34
    techniques 55ff.
Greater sphenoid wing 12

H
Hess chart 27

I
Immediate surgery, contraindications 30
Inferior orbital fissure 3
Internal orbital fractures 10
    materials for repair of 34

K
Key area
   definition 2
   reconstruction 58

L
Lacrimal duct injuries 53
Landmarks, for reduction of the zygoma 49
Linear fractures (see Internal orbital fractures)
Lower eyelid incision 44

M
Marginotomies 45
Mask lift techniques (see Soft tissue resuspension)
Materials, for repair of internal orbital
   fractures 34
Mid-eyelid incision (see Lower eyelid incision)
Motility disorder
   management 27
   mechanical 24
   neurogenic 26

O
Optic canal fracture 24
Optic nerve
   decompression in the canal 23
   enlargement of sheet 22
Orbital floor fractures (see Blow-out fractures)
Orbital frame   2
   inner 38
   outer 78
Orbital plate (see Rigid fixation)
Orbital pyramid 2
Orbital septae 3

P
PDS sheet 55f.
Posterior medial wall (see Key area)

R
RAPD (relative afferent pupillary defect) 20
Restrictive motility disorder 24
Retrobulbar hematoma 18, 22
Retrobulbar pain 14
Revision surgery 39
Rigid fixation
   for internal orbital fractures 55f.
   systems 47
ROA (rapid ophthalmic assessment) 20

S
Segmental reconstruction 55
Soft tissue
   sagging 48
   resuspension 48
Subciliary incision 44
Steroids (see Corticosteroids)
Superior orbital fissure, syndrome 12
Swinging flash light test 21

T
Telecanthus, correction of 76
Temporal hollowing 36, 78
Titanium 47
Transnasal canthopexy (see Canthopexy)
Traumatic optic neuropathy 21

U
Upper blepharoplasty incision 44
Upper buccal sulcus incision 44

V
Visual loss
   management 22
   mechanisms 18, 33
Visibility, enhancement of 55

W
Waters view 13

Z
Zygomatic arch, as landmark 51